Illusion of the Body

Introducing the Body Alive Principle

David Almeida

Illusion of the Body

Acknowledgements

I would like to express my sincere appreciation to those who helped make this book possible:

To the Divine Source for making this journey possible
To my wife, a life coach, for her amazing courage
To her wonderful family for always being there
To my mother and father for their giving all they've got
To my brother and sisters for giving me pleasant memories
To all of my friends for their encouragement
To all those who has contributed to my happiness over the years
Special thanks to Sarah for her significant contribution
I'd also like to extend my thanks to my editors and publisher

DISCLAIMER

This book details the author's personal experiences with and opinions about alternative medicine. The author is not a health care provider.

The author and publisher are providing this book and its contents on an "as is" basis and make no representations or warranties of any kind with respect to this book or its contents. The author and publisher disclaim all such representations and warranties, including, for example, warranties of merchantability and health care for a particular purpose. In addition, the author and publisher do not represent or warrant that the information accessible via this book is accurate, complete or current.

The statements made about products and services have not been evaluated by the U.S. Food and Drug Administration. They are not intended to diagnose, treat, cure, or prevent any condition or disease. Please consult with your own physician or healthcare professional regarding the suggestions and recommendations made in this book.

Except as specifically stated in this book, neither the author or publisher, nor any authors, contributors, or other representatives will be liable for damages arising out of or in connection with the use of this book. This is a comprehensive limitation of liability that applies to all damages of any kind, including (without limitation) compensatory; direct, indirect or consequential damages; loss of data, income or profit; loss of or damage to property and claims of third parties.

You understand that this book is not intended as a substitute for consultation with a licensed health care practitioner, such as your physician. Before you begin any health care program, or change your lifestyle in any way, you will consult your physician or other licensed healthcare practitioner to ensure that you are in good health and that the examples contained in this book will not harm you.

This book provides content related to topics on physical and/or mental health issues. As such, use of this book implies your acceptance of this disclaimer.

Table of Contents

Introducing the Body Alive Principle

PART I

Introduction

"You only live once, but if you do it right, once is enough."
Mae West

I almost cannot recall where the inspiration for this book came from, although it undoubtedly originated with the Divine Source. Although, I can say I have had a longtime fascination with consciousness. What is it? Where does it reside? How did it come to be? At some point, I came to realize that I not only exist in my body as a sentient being but that my whole world is alive. This means the physical world as I define it. I came to learn that matter, in its many forms, has its own intelligence and awareness. This is a philosophy known as panpsychism. From this philosophy, I extracted panpsychic healing. Panpsychic healing is at the heart of what I call the Body Alive Principle. This is the idea that the body is a legion of conscious entities, from the organs right down to the cells and their atoms. I refer to these entities as the "little minds." That is the first concept behind the Body Alive Principle. The second part of this theory asserts that the mind can heal the body by instructing the body's internal structures and cells to do just that. Positive self-talk or affirmative language can achieve this end.

I make use of Maslow's hierarchy of needs pyramid to discuss human needs and the needs of the body. Because our mind and bodies are intimately connected, a mutually dependent relationship exists between the two. The needs of the human mind or "super mind" have

9

a strong effect on the needs of the little minds, and vice versa. This relationship is comparable to the need for food and shelter, and the need for self-actualization. This subject is one of the most pertinent ideas put forward in this text. Understanding human needs will bestow a comprehension that may seem like a shortcut to traditional learning. This knowledge will help you to implement the tools of the Body Alive Principle.

I, like most people, have family and friends with serious illnesses. The idea for the Body Alive Principal came to me as a desire to provide permanent relief to those living with debilitating illnesses. Many people believe that the mind can heal the body, and there is plenty of evidence to back up that notion. Most people do not realize that their body pays attention to what they think. Not only is that statement true, but it's also true that the body will act on these unconscious messages. This is true of both the positive and negative messages that we send it. For example, if you say, "I feel good!" (Thank you, James Brown), your body will respond by producing feel-good chemicals such as endorphins. If you say, "I feel terrible!" Your body will then create illness. Yes, this is a deliberate act of your body responding to your subconscious commands. This idea is vital to the Body Alive Principle.

The body will also send messages to you when something is not right. This commonly comes in the form of pain, fatigue, nausea, headaches, dizziness, etc. You can see that there is a constant mental dialogue going on between you and your body. While this is not a startling revelation in itself, it takes on a new dimension when you consider that your body is alive. The good news is that you can consciously communicate with the zillions of cellular entities that make your earthly journey possible. Communication with your body is initiated in several ways. Of these techniques, the most effective are creative visualization and positive affirmations. These are powerful tools for providing direction to your body. They are fundamental to the Body Alive Principle.

Creative visualization, using our powerful imagination, is one process that is drawn on to make positive changes in the body. *Guided imagery* is the act of assisting another person in using his or her imagination, as hypnotists do. Visualization is a powerful tool in the arsenal of the Body Alive Principle. The application of affirmative language in conjunction with visualization ensures that the little minds will receive your messages. A number of other popular complementary therapies make use of both techniques. The Body Alive Principle makes use of them in a unique way. Throughout this book, I will encourage you to continue your studies by reading other books on the various topics I present. This book is by no means the authority on visualization or affirmations. This is also true of the following techniques that I mention.

Another valuable technique covered in this book is *empathetic listening*. This skill requires the listener to remain closely engaged with the other party, and to do so without interrupting or forming opinions that will impede the process. Empathetic listening teaches us to pay attention, which is extremely important when it comes to the body. Our bodies are constantly sending us operational signals. Some of these messages are obvious, and others are rather subtle. Recognizing these signals can save us from future pain. You will learn how to put empathetic listening to use in developing a better relationship with other people and your body.

Mindfulness meditation is another tool this book will explore. Mindfulness also teaches us to pay attention. Like many meditation practices, there is a desire to quiet the mind. Inevitably, we learn to slow down our racing thoughts. This helps us to receive those intuitive messages from the little minds. While any meditation practice is helpful in achieving this state, mindfulness is especially useful in expanding our awareness of our body, including breathing, sound, physical sensations, and thoughts. Mindfulness is a key component of the Body Alive Principle since the little minds need our attention to do their jobs. You will have a better understanding of mindfulness meditation, including how it relates to the Body Alive Principle, after reading through that portion of the book.

There are also separate sections for dealing with both guilt and trauma. Guilt's relationship to the Body Alive Principle is in need of its own attention. Poor health leads directly to the door of guilt. It even has a welcome mat. I have created my own five-step process for conquering this difficult emotion. Trauma is of immense concern to all healers. Many of the worst health problems experienced in the modern era have their origin in traumas.

One fundamental aspect of the Body Alive Principle is living with integrity in order to bring your body into balance. The positive attributes, discussed in this book, are honesty, **trust, kindness, empathy, gentleness, self-control, and** integrity. These desirable qualities are the key to our continued well-being. If you do your best to maintain these qualities, you will increase the likelihood of a long and healthy life. Our bodies require us to operate with these precious qualities in order to maintain homeostasis. This book reminds us that, although we will never reach a definite point of perfection in our character, we must always strive to improve ourselves by doing our best to conduct our personal affairs with these qualities in mind.

I have learned that there are resources beyond our understanding ready to assist us in reaching our goals. This includes the cosmic consciousness, which some call God. The Body Alive Principle may be exactly what you need, where nothing else has worked. The truth is that we all need to be in touch with our bodies for obvious reasons. The primary reason is that we cannot manage life's journey without it. As many have said, we have one body in this lifetime. If we do not take care of it, it will not take care of us. To have a better experience in the physical world, we need to ensure that we treat the body with respect and understanding, as with all things we love.

My motivation in writing this book is to pass on what the higher forces have revealed to me for the benefit of others, particularly those who are stuck in a rut, sick, anxious, depressed, lonely, angry, resentful, or bitter. My intention is to alleviate and ultimately end suffering. I realize people experience pain for many reasons, and some will not respond to any medical treatment. Sometimes people do not want their conditions healed because they harbor guilt. Other people choose their afflictions before coming into this world. However for those of you who truly desire healing, the Body Alive Principle makes it possible. By developing the skills presented in this book, and with a little patience, you will have an excellent opportunity to heal yourself or someone else.

I want to add that this book is not a scholarly or academic work. It is a metaphysical work, that I feel cannot be properly judged by those claiming superior academic intelligence. The Body Alive Principle deals with ideas that are foreign to us. Therefore, *current* methods of scientific examination will not be able to determine its mechanism. This is also the case with alternative therapies such as reiki and acupuncture. However, I will endeavor to present reasonable data to support my claims. I have attempted to access suitable websites with quality information. It's likely that some of these web pages will be gone years from now. That's not a problem. You will find that the integrity of this publication has a solid foundation. My main concern is that my readers learn something valuable from this book. I implore you to keep an open mind and use this book in faith. Science only accounts for a small fraction of what takes place in our universe. Our knowledge of reality is truly incomplete.

The Body Alive Principle: What You Need to Know

"Everything you can imagine is real."
Pablo Picasso

What is Panpsychism?

My definition of panpsychism is that it is an ancient philosophy that all things, both animate and inanimate, have consciousness and awareness. This includes all animal, vegetable, and mineral entities. There are opposing views among practicing panpsychists in regards to what qualifies as consciousness, as well as which inanimate objects are eligible for the panpsychic designation. I believe that all material things have consciousness. I also believe that many levels of consciousness exist to which we are intricately connected. Some of the major systems include:

- The body with its individual cells, organs, and systems

- Our higher or greater self

- The mass mind, which is the Collective Consciousness of all living humans

- The Earth itself, which is a living organism with its own unique systems and mechanisms

- The Infinite Intelligence, or God, to which all
  things are connected

Consciousness is not limited to living and inanimate entities. It also includes thoughts and emotions. All mental structures have their own awareness and personalities. Thoughts compete with one another to manifest into reality. They race to the surface, much like sperm race to infuse with the egg (I hope you don't mind the analogy). Emotions do much the same, fighting to be the dominant mental state. They are energetic beings and are alive like anything else.

I should point out that panpsychism is unrelated to fortune telling or any other crystal ball gazing phenomena, although I'm not condemning any practitioners of this craft. My goal is to help others live better lives.

What is the Body Alive Principle and how does it work?

This is a unique healing system, which does not require invasive drugs, surgeries, or expensive treatments. The Body Alive Principle is the art of communicating with the sentient beings comprising our bodies, to bring relief from disease.

Your body does all of the healing, together with the aid of your exceptional leadership. I am of the opinion that the mind is separate from the body. I believe our bodies are organic containers meant to sustain our spiritual selves – an organism comprised of millions of separate entities that make physical life possible. This goes against the popular, scientific belief that the mind is a function of the brain.

The Body Alive Principle promotes the idea that our internal structures are alive with their own consciousness just like ours. In other words, they have their own unique personalities and have their own experiences taking place. In years past, people attributed human qualities to organs. For instance, many countries have designated the heart as the center of love.

As I said, this idea moves right down to the very cells of the body. Each entity must answer to the super mind for direction. So the cells must report to the organs, and the whole body must report to us. Thus, we are the super mind and the ultimate authority. The body needs direction, or it will take matters into its own hands. No pun intended. If something is going wrong with our bodies, it is because they are receiving these messages from us. This mix up *can be* from trauma existing in the subconscious. There are many other reasons for disease. Communicating with our bodies in an effective way can often alleviate these medical problems. The Body Alive Principle uses creative visualization, an optimistic attitude, and positive language/commands to communicate with the little minds. In many cases, this practice can provide lasting relief for even the worst medical conditions.

The other part is learning how to respond to your bodily needs. Your body has needs just like all living things. If you neglect those needs, you risk acquiring any number of human diseases. Your body will make you aware of their needs. An example of this is fatigue. It's the body's signal for us to slow down. It's a remarkably strong signal. Many of the things your body needs may not seem obvious, but they are usually the same things you require to feel well.

Is the Body Alive Principle a New Age Concept?

I do not believe that the Body Alive Principle is comparable to other healing practices in use at this time. I feel it stands on its own as both a healing therapy and a way of life. Panpsychism is a distinct theory of mind. This philosophy has earned the respect of spiritually aware people, belonging to some the world's greatest civilizations, for thousands of years. The finer points of panpsychism can be located in any good philosophical text. I want to point out, that other healing practices, such as hypnosis, also employ the techniques advanced by the Body Alive Principle. I am not claiming to offer any new ideas in that regard. I am just bringing a forgotten healing art back into the light. I originally created the Body Alive Principle as a hypnosis script, which I intended to use as a method for treating my wife's autoimmune disorders.

Since I had already accepted the panpsychic theory, I thought I might apply it to the human body. This process also prompted me to obtain my certification as a hypnotist. We had success with this technique, where only Prednisone (a nasty drug as far as side effects go) was helping to manage her illness. My wife's change in awareness also changed her relationship with her body. She began treating her body as the multi-conscious complex organism it is. She learned to meditate and communicate effectively with her body. The Body Alive Principle was instrumental in improving her condition. She leads a full and active life despite these medical intrusions. Please understand that results will vary from person to person. The good news is that this is something we can all do.

Why isn't there a systematic process for the Body Alive Principle?

I realize everyone wants a paint-by-numbers approach to any alternative healing technique. I do not believe a systematic process is necessary to implement the Body Alive Principle. Your success with this practice has more to do with awareness and attitude than working an actual system; at least as we tend to think of it. The instructions given in this book, such as problem solving and living with integrity are transformational. They are at the very heart of the Body Alive Principle. This practice eventually becomes a way of life.

The Body Alive Principle uses time-honored healing methods to achieve communication with the inner structures of our bodies. There is nothing new about the modalities used in this book. I'm talking about meditation, creative visualization, empathetic listening, and other practices used to activate the Body Alive Principle. Anyone with an average imagination can master these modalities. The information contained in this book is straightforward, and anyone with enough motivation can make it work. This book clearly outlines the action steps needed to be successful with the practical applications. If there is a request for it, I would be willing to design a training curriculum to encourage its acceptance.

How do I know if it is working for me?

If you see any relief from your symptoms, it may be a sign that exercising a panpsychic mind is positively affecting your life. Only you know how you feel and whether your condition is improving. Even waking up in a better mood may be an indication that the Body Alive Principle is benefitting you. You should carefully conduct a thorough self-examination of your current physical and mental state, and compare it to what your condition was prior to employing the techniques in this book. You will "know" inside whether or not this is working for you.

These are some questions you might ask yourself to determine your current physical condition:

- Am I experiencing frequent headaches?
- Do I have back pain?
- Is there any other persistent pain in my body?
- Do I feel dizzy at times?
- Have I had diarrhea or vomiting for more than a few days?
- Do I have shortness of breath?
- Do I experience an upset stomach?
- Have I been fighting a lingering cold?
- Do I have a cough that won't go away?
- Do I have a sore throat that will not go away?
- Am I feeling any weakness in my limbs?
- Is my temperature running high or low?
- Has my weight gone up or down dramatically in a short time?
- Do I feel overly anxious?
- Have I been depressed for a long time?

There are many other symptom-related questions you could ask yourself in order to get an accurate picture of your current physical condition. The symptoms listed here may be common to your diagnosis, and you will certainly know which ones are applicable. Some of these symptoms have specific criteria. For instance, when you have been feeling sad, or hopelessness, for a period of two weeks or more, doctors may diagnose depression. At least, I'm told this is one of the criteria doctors use. As I said, you will know whether certain symptoms are common to your illness. I don't think there is any need for me to venture into the details of medical science. I'm sure the medical professionals would prefer I didn't.

After determining your current state of health, you will be able, with accuracy, to assess your initial progress with the Body Alive

Principle. Credit for any improvement in your condition, may be given, at least in part, to the Body Alive Principle. Of course, you should also consider any other lifestyle changes you have made during this time. Even if you do not know what to attribute your improvement to, I would suggest you continue using the Body Alive Principle for good measure.

How long do I have to work the Body Alive Principle before I see results?

There is no real time frame for obtaining results with this practice. Your enthusiasm will get you there quicker. However, this process may take a bit longer depending upon the outside factors involved. I advise that you practice daily and give this lost treatment a fair chance to prove itself. It will be worth it.

Should I stop my current medical treatment to pursue this system?

I cannot advise you as to whether or not you should continue to work with your medical providers. I do not recommend that you suddenly stop any treatment, regardless of the results you are getting from the Body Alive Principle. I do not want anyone to come to harm by going against his or her physician's advice. Please use discretion in making such decisions. In most cases, the Body Alive Principle can enhance your current medical treatment plan. I believe that it can be just as effective on its own. In any case, it's recommended that you gradually introduce the Body Alive Principle into your treatment plan. You may wish to continue this way if you see improvement.

Is the Body Alive Principle for me?

Only you can answer that question. I believe that everyone should have a close relationship with his or her body. Everyone should want to be healthy in body, mind, and spirit. Our bodies are working hard for us, so we should take an interest in what is going on with them. The body we were given is the only one we will have in this lifetime. Sometimes it's necessary to look at things differently in order to make positive changes. The Body Alive Principle works for anyone with any known illness. There are different levels of success with this technique, which range from mild to outstanding. It's different for everyone. The only way you will know if this practice is for you is to try it out.

Philosophy of Panpsychism

My definition of panpsychism is that all things have independent minds and are part of the Universal Mind. Panpsychism is a form of idealism. Without getting into a complicated discourse on idealism, let's say that it is the view that reality is mentally based. Idealism is the belief that we live in a "mentalverse". It states that all things exist mentally.

Idealism opposes the idea of materialism or physicalism, which is the belief that the universe consists solely of matter. This theory states that the universe is physical. It makes for a compelling argument, since we are able to perceive the material world through our five senses, whereas the mentalverse is hard to locate and define. Related to physicalism is realism, which advocates the belief that things exist independently of the mind. This philosophy specifies that the outside world has absolute existence.

Idealism and materialism both ascribe to a philosophy called monism. Monism supposes that the universe is made of a single substance. Here, you might say one atom is the same as another. Everything is made of the same basic material. Monism enthusiasts believe that the universe and everything in it exists as a single unit. This is the "we are one" factor. We are all part of the machine. Nothing is independent of the whole. It is also the idea that the physical and nonphysical are but one substance. There is no division between the two. Monism is the opposite of dualism, which says that the universe is made of two substances. This statement includes mind and matter. Dualism creates a distinct line between the physical and nonphysical.

There are several theories related to panpsychism:

Panexperientialism holds that all entities possess consciousness, but without any level of intelligence as we know it.

Panprotoexperientialism says that entities do possess consciousness, but have neither intelligence nor awareness of their own existence.

Animism is a philosophical or spiritual belief that certain nonphysical objects and forces possess souls or spirits. This includes (but is not limited to) animals, plants, minerals, and weather phenomenon, as well as land and water features.

Hylozoism is a philosophy that proposes that some things possess life, and regards life and matter to have an inherent connection.

Pantheism is a philosophy that promotes the idea that there is no distinction between God and creation. Pantheists believe "God" and the universe to be one complete unit. You could say God is in the mix.

There are too many forms of idealism to mention here. Philosophy goes off in many directions and has many flavors. If you are interested in this subject, I encourage you to explore it for yourself. It is great for personal growth. Just don't lose yourself in the process.

Big minds and the little minds

Rest your hand in your lap or on some other surface and then lift it up to scratch your head. How did your hand know to do that? This is a clear example of how your mind produced a signal, processed by your brain, to command your hand to do that. It's a remarkable feat, and something we never stop to consider. It establishes the fact that the mind commands the body.

The mind controls bodily functions that are extremely sensitive, like breathing and tissue repair. Many of these processes are automatic. We're not even aware of their magnificent works. It's fascinating to those in the know that we are not burdened with the details of running our own bodies. As the super minds (I don't mean that in an egotistical way), we're allowed to dwell on matters that we feel are of far greater importance, such as what we'll be eating for dinner or what we're going to wear to work the next day.

It's like being the president. Although we run the whole show, we honestly don't know what everyone below us is doing. We have to put our faith in the system. We trust that we have hired the right people to do the job. As far as the body goes, the job always gets done in the best possible way.

Sometimes we're born with certain conditions like diabetes, cystic fibrosis, mental illness, or other compromising medical illnesses. This presents a challenge to the system. Our employees, which we know as the little minds, now have to work harder. That's fine – they can deal with it. They're willing to work overtime to make the organization successful. You will find it advantageous to have these guys on your team. If you were able to see what's going on in your body, you would probably appreciate them a little more. Our employees make the company what it is. They are its assets.

I want to point out that not only are we able to command the cells and organs of our bodies, we are able to manage the multitudes of bacteria that exist within us, as well. They will listen to our mental instructions. We are capable of turning the most notorious germs into harmless or even beneficial roommates. Do I think this is an easy task? I would say no, but that is why you should practice the exercises in this book. Part of the process is developing the right attitude, as you will see.

Our bodies will do what it takes. We have a tendency to take our bodies for granted. It's not until we suddenly lose our precious health, that we pull up a chair and take notice. We might say, "How did this happen to me! This is terrible!" It shows how little we understand our own bodies. That's not a sarcastic remark. As a rule, our bodies run so well that we don't even give it a thought. Because of this, complacency has become quite common about personal health and wellness.

Nothing more than feelings

Emotion affects all things and goes beyond our current understanding. Emotion is universal. Emotions excite cells and atoms. Without feelings, we would certainly be lifeless. I have a theory that the main reason we decide to come into this life is to experience emotion. Emotion puts the world *in motion*. It's clear to me that all living and "non-living" entities have emotion. I can hear you saying, "Oh man is this guy one slice short of a loaf!" I realize this is a difficult concept to take in. Has anyone ever seriously entertained the idea of a rock having emotion? The name given to the practice of attributing human qualities to inanimate objects is *pathetic* or *anthropomorphic fallacy*. This ancient practice became an imaginative writer's tool in literature called "personification". This is an age-old belief that goes back (as far we can trace) to ancient Greece. I can recall cartoons from my childhood that featured inanimate objects dancing and singing. Don't get me wrong - I'm not saying your dinnerware and silverware are going to get up and do the conga. I'm not the first to propose the panpsychic theory. However, I believe I'm the first to do so publicly; at least in recent times.

I do not know to what extent "things" feel. When your car breaks down on the highway, and you kick it and call it stupid, can you hurt its feelings? I'm not talking about Herbie the Love Bug. Even if I could say so, how would I go about proving it using *current* scientific methods? That's not an easy task in this day and age. The answer to the equation comes down to an inner knowing that anyone can possess. You may not have psychic powers, or meditate on a mountaintop all day, but you can still feel the truth. Just a walk in the woods or by the ocean will allow you to hear the voices and feel the love. You will enjoy unrestricted access to this secret world if both your heart and mind are open.

Even lacking evidence that things have feelings, I do believe we should handle our possessions with care. They may not tolerate abuse. What happens to your car when you don't do the routine maintenance? It breaks down. Is it a stretch to say that it broke down because you didn't care about it? Not necessarily. It does take an adjustment in our thinking to see it this way. You have to look at the nature of things differently. Let's just say this makes for a better quality of life.

Some have said that physical objects form an uncanny attachment to their owners. Have you ever heard stories of people who have lost valuable and sentimental objects such as jewelry, only to find them far away? Or perhaps a stranger returns them to the owner. Maybe this has happened to you. It can seem supernatural. It's an intriguing thought from my perspective. It's like the cat that came back the very next day. Our possessions have an emotional bond with us. This usually happens because we have a special attachment to our objects. Love is pervasive. It is the sole quality of the Universal Mind that is present everywhere, all the time. Every atom, cell, and structure understands this premise.

If we took care of our belongings, as our wise parents should have taught us, we would have a much better relationship with the things in our environment. I agree with those who say that we're a throwaway society. When we have lost all interest in an object, we quickly throw it away without a second thought. Some of us have flagrant disregard for the things in our lives that truly matter. When we begin to change our attitude toward material objects, our interpersonal relationships with one another are likely to change, as well.

A suggestion would be that you reuse or recycle your belongings. Would you like to make some extra cash? Of course, you would. Why not sell your unwanted items rather than throw them away? You could even donate your stuff. Articles that you can donate include furniture, clothing, books, and just about anything else. By doing this, you will put yourself in the right frame of mind to understand what I am talking about.

We should consider the feelings of all things whether we can sense their life or not. Yes, I am an extreme panpsychist. I believe our five senses are not sophisticated enough to comprehend what is happening all around us. When we are young, adults teach us the mantra, "I'll believe it when I see it." Well, I'm sorry, just because you can't see it, doesn't mean it isn't there. That would rule out the existence of x-rays, ultraviolet, infrared, and gamma rays. What can we say about those extremely high and low sounds that escape our ears, the ones that are inaudible? What would our world look like if we could fully experience it? That's a question best left to the professional metaphysicists.

PART II

The Evidence

"Facts do not cease to exist because they are ignored."
Aldous Huxley (Complete Essays 2, 1926-29)

The philosophy behind panpsychism and the Body Alive Principle may seem implausible. That is to be expected. Our understanding of reality is incomplete. As I discussed earlier, our five senses are crude and give us a limited, or even skewed, view of reality. For the most part, the only humans who can provide an accurate account of reality are those people who have transitioned to the other side.

An analytical mind such as that of an investigator, engineer, or medical professional will have the most trouble accepting panpsychic healing. I am sure the Body Alive Principle qualifies as metaphysics. Many people immediately disregard anything having to do with metaphysics because it does not conform to the conventional rules of science. It lies beyond what is known or empirically provable. Using traditional methods of inquiry, we come up short.

Consciousness is indefinable. The essence of consciousness cannot be isolated in a test tube. Still, we are able to detect certain pieces of our true nature at times. It's like looking at a massive machine that produces reality and only being able to see small parts of it at one time. As the saying goes, "God only gives us what we can handle." I believe consciousness can only handle one thought or action at a time – at least in physical reality. If we could view the master plan, our heads would explode. In the paragraphs that follow, I present the works of several historical personalities that I believe will add weight to the body alive principle as well as the idea of a collective consciousness.

Cellular Memory

Cellular memory is the idea that the cells of the human body each contain a complete record of our experiential history from the time we are born. Proponents of the cellular memory theory (including myself) state that this information includes memories, interests, habits, tastes, and more. The cellular memory theory rests on the stories of organ transplant recipients who received publicity for acquiring the memories and personal traits of their donors.

In the 1970s, a woman named Claire Sylvia received a heart-lung transplant from an 18-year old donor who had been in a motorcycle accident. Sylvia began exhibiting unusual tastes and habits post-operatively. She began having cravings for beer and foods she had never eaten prior to the transplant. Sylvia wrote an account of her extraordinary experience in a book called *A Change of Heart.* In 2002, her story became a television movie entitled "Heart of a Stranger," starring Jane Seymour. This movie seems to be hard to find, but you could check out your local video store. There are other cases not mentioned here that are probably worth investigating. Most of them are not celebrity cases, however. The Discovery Health Channel delved into the remarkable world of cellular memory in a program titled "Transplanting Memories." The show presents actual cases of this phenomenon. I refer you to this website for additional information: http://perdurabo10.tripod.com/id470.html.

We know that the DNA molecules, which make up the genes in our chromosomes, carry the blueprints for genetic inheritance. When cell division takes place, an exact copy of the dividing cell is formed containing the exact components needed to build another cell; this includes proteins and RNA molecules. Through DNA and gene cloning, we are able to reproduce a complete copy of the original organism. In the same way that human cells carry genetic information when they divide, the cells also contain the personal qualities, habits, mannerisms, and other traits that make up the organism. Cells also transfer memories of every kind, including sensations such as those coming through our five senses. Although there is no rational explanation for why this occurs, my metaphysical theory is that all cells in a single body have access to the same information. They are all one. Although they are independent, they are part of the whole. I believe that you can see this in ants and bees. I guess you could say it's a group mentality. Yes, that's very true. Everything you've ever experienced is contained in each one of your cells and even their atoms. I don't know what the mechanism is behind this process. Scientists have not given cellular awareness the attention it deserves. So, for now its secret will remain a mystery.

George De La Warr and Radionics

In the 1950s, a British inventor named George De La Warr developed an area of psychic research known as radionics, a field of study that came into existence in the early 1900s through the research of Albert Abrams. Radionics bases its efficacy on the idea that each person has unique frequencies. Some frequencies indicate health and others disease. In his experiments to find practical applications for his radionic equipment, De La Warr concluded that each cell is capable of transmitting a unique electrical charge to another part of itself. Therefore, a cell can also transmit many invisible qualities unique to that cell, including its distinct energy patterns. De La Warr invented devices, a camera in particular, which he claimed would register these energy patterns. He declared that this special camera could do nothing less than detect and cure diseases from a distance. De la Warr claimed that these devices registered a radiation pattern that could display the appearance and composition of the tissue under examination. With a suitable tissue sample, the camera would amazingly reveal the organism's pathology. I'll also note that a civil claim was filed against De La Warr in 1960. The litigant was a woman named Catherine Phillips. Philips claimed De La Warr's diagnostic device led to her ill health. I'm not too concerned about these civil suits since people can sue for any reason, even if there is no merit to their complaint.

De La Warr founded De La Warr Laboratories in order to build his devices. From what I can tell, the company operated in relative obscurity until 1987, In fact, De La Warr's original radionic devices and related paraphernalia have since vanished without a trace.

De La Warr's research with human frequencies shows that we each carry unique vibrations. These vibrations emanate from one source. It's like being part of a group with a common vision, while retaining our own personal ambitions. One atom is the same as another atom, but each is one of a kind. It's something of a contradiction, but I'm sure that you get my point.[1, 2]

Dr. Harold Saxon Burr and L-fields

It was a Massachusetts native, Dr. Harold Saxton Burr (1889-1973), a Professor of Anatomy at the Yale University School of

Medicine, who coined the term *L-fields* or *life fields* to describe the electrodynamic fields that he hypothesized to be the blueprints of every living creature. "Note that the word "living" was a highly subjective one to Dr. Burr. Dr. Burr measured and mapped these invisible fields of vitality through his unconventional use of a voltmeter. Dr. Burr employed this instrument to study the bioelectric qualities of menstruation, ovulation, and cancer, among other things. Most notable, among his experiments are the ones performed on the salamander and frog eggs. Starting with the salamander specimen, he proceeded to mark the peak voltage on the egg. As the embryos developed, the peak voltage never changed. However, it turned out to be located at the creature's head. Dr. Burr theorized that the greatest voltage point was the blueprint for the arrangement of the salamander's fully-grown nervous system. Dr. Burr then repeated this experiment on frog eggs and came to the same conclusion. Dr. Burr held that L-fields also directed mental and emotional states. He maintained that their activity was evident using his instruments. These experiments seemed to show that the L-fields are the organizing force behind the creation of life. Dr. Burr disregarded the idea of a vital or universal life force. He was content to study and develop the idea of a controlling human energetic force. In spite of this, Burr's L-fields lend credence to the presence of divine consciousness orchestrating the design of life. [3, 4]

Jagdish Chandra Bose

Dr. Bose was born in 1858 in Mymensingh, Bengal. In 1884, he received a B.Sc from the University of London. On his return in 1885, Bose became a professor of physics at Presidency College in Calcutta. Bose faced serious challenges from his English colleagues. It seems they did not approve of an Indian joining their ranks. Bose was offered a salary half that of his colleagues. True to his character, Bose took things in stride and stayed in the game. Bose has many supporters who consider him as the true "Father of Wireless Telegraphy". In 1894, Bose unveiled this extraordinary technology to the public. He was able to demonstrate to a large audience how radio waves could travel through a wall 75 feet away and ring a bell. Shortly thereafter, the Italian inventor Guglielmo Marconi was able to construct a device that generated radio waves, for which he obtained a patent, and became known as the official father of wireless technology.

What is particularly relevant to this book is the research that Bose conducted in biology. Bose was perhaps the first reputable scientist of his day, to declare that plants and metals are alive in the truest sense. Bose publicly announced that plants feel pain and express affection. He believed that plants have a central nervous system that responds to shock in the same way an animal does. Bose also concluded that plants thrive when exposed to soothing music, as opposed to harsh noise. Over the years, researchers have arrived at similar results to those of Bose.

In 1906, Bose published the all-important monograph, "Response in The Living and Nonliving." This research paper revealed that plant and animal tissue share a comparable electric impulse response to all manner of stimuli. He was even able to show that certain rocks and metals have these same responses to stimulation. Bose also discovered that the life force in metals could be impaired or eliminated altogether when subjected to electrical stimulation and pressure. In Bose's experiments with scissors and small machinery, he found that they eventually experience fatigue. The objects were able to regain lost energy through rest. One could easily construe the results of Bose's experiments to mean that metals have consciousness, and perhaps even memories.

The idea that plants and metals are alive was a revolutionary one to promote at that time and place. However, Bose managed to gain the respect of the Royal Society for his commendable efforts. In 1920, the Royal Society elected Bose to the esteemed position of fellow. Prior to his death in 1937, the Bose Institute at Calcutta was established. I'd like to encourage you to do a little research on this underappreciated historical figure. He was truly fascinating.[5, 6, 7]

The Backster Effect

Cleve Backster is a professional polygraphist and the owner of the Backster School of Lie Detection, founded in New York City. The school is now located in San Diego, California. Most associate Backster's name with his famous plant experiments in the 1960s. Backster first stumbled onto the idea of "primary perception" (as he coined it) in plants when, out of curiosity, he hooked a galvanometer up to a corn plant to see how long it would take for water poured on the plant roots, to reach its leaves. To his surprise, the graph paper showed a downward trend. Backster took this to mean that the corn plant was giving feedback indicating pleasurable stimulation. Backster then proceeded to take this in the other direction and tried dunking a leaf in hot coffee. There was no reaction. Then Backster contemplated burning the leaf. Before Backster could move to take action on the flaming image in his mind, the machine recorded a long upward progression. Many admirers of Backster's work take this event to mean the corn plant could read his thoughts.

Backster has conducted hundreds of experiments in an effort to support this unique theory. One of these experiments showed that a plant attuned to its caretaker, could read that person's thought from a considerable distance. This means a common house plant can connect to a caretaker's emotional signals, such as when he is in danger.

Backster discovered additional evidence at the cellular level. One of Backster's plants reacted to his eating a cup of yogurt. Backster realized the jam he was adding to the yogurt contained a chemical that was killing the yogurt's bacteria. This unexplained event happened again when Backster cut his finger and applied iodine. Backster finally identified the cause of the polygraph's striking pattern when he observed the plants were reacting to hot water poured down a sink, which was killing the bacteria in it. Apparently, the plant was reacting to the death of the microbes. Associates of Backster thought that some form of "cellular consciousness" was at work.

Backster devised an automated test that involved dropping brine shrimp into a pot of boiling water. The response from the three Heart Leaf Philodendrons attached to galvanometers demonstrated their sensitivity to the death of the shrimp. This experiment showed results similar to those of the previously mentioned incidents. It supports the cellular consciousness theory. Backster's experiments raised the attention of the media. This fascination changed the way that people see plant life.

The Secret Life of Plants, by Peter Tompkins and Christopher Bird, quoted Backster as saying, "Sentience does not seem to stop at the cellular level. It may go down all the way to the molecular, the atomic, and even the subatomic level. All sorts of objects which have traditionally been considered to be inanimate may have to be re-evaluated."

During these trials, Backster coined the term "primary perception", which theorizes the existence of a field that connects all living things and is outside the realm of our five senses. However, it exists independent of extra-sensory perception.

One of my favorite researchers happens to be. Not only do I appreciate Backster for his substantial contribution to metaphysics, I also admire him for his unorthodox and controversial methods. I love it when science is unable to comprehend something that exists and operates outside of conventional thinking.

The Secret Life of Plants by Peter Tompkins and Christopher Bird is an excellent information source on Backster, and the other unconventional researchers in this section. This publication's well-written account, of the accomplishments of these little-known researchers, prompted me to conduct further research into their fascinating lives. I suggest that the book I just mentioned, along with the websites I list in the footnotes, would be an excellent place to start. You may also want to check out, *Primary Perception: Biocommunication with Plants, Living Food, and Human Cells,* by Cleve Backster himself.[8, 9, 10]

PART III

What the Body Needs

"Do your own thing on your own terms and get what you came here for."
Oliver James

The Hustle and Bustle

In America, we are extremely out of touch with our inner being. We're so busy being busy that we don't take the time to tend to our personal needs. The average person goes from one task to the next without taking a breath. As humans living in modern society, we have obligations. These obligations include our family, job, and various other people and groups. We have to take care of these responsibilities. We can avoid these things, but we leave ourselves open to being labeled as irresponsible. Is this unfair? I don't know. It depends on the nature of the obligation. Making sure our children eat meals everyday is easy to judge. On the other hand, holding an extravagant party for your child's baseball team may be unnecessary, especially if it strains you.

You have to set your priorities. In the grand scheme of things, building a birdhouse for your grandmother does not usually qualify as a critical project, although it is a kind act of love. We all have the same amount of time to work with. It's up to us to decide how to use it. Sometimes, as kindhearted people, we feel we're being selfish for not fulfilling everyone's requests. It's as if we're disappointing those we love for not coming through on every request or favor asked of us. This isn't fair to us. We overextend ourselves trying to meet every demand that comes our way.

I'm not trying to discount anyone's needs. We all know people in our lives that depend on the services of others for their existence, including children and sometimes the elderly. We are responsible for their needs. However, their needs cannot come before our own vital needs. I like the example of the mother with her little child next to her on a plane that has just encountered some difficulty. The captain tells the passengers to put on their oxygen masks. The mother's immediate reaction is to place the child's mask on first. This is the wrong thing to do. Why? If the mother passes out, she will not be able to help her child or herself. It is important for the mother to put her own mask on first and then tend to her child. I certainly understand the mother's instinct.

You have to take care of your needs first. It isn't because you are being mean or negligent. It's natural to care about the needs of your family and friends. However, it's necessary to take care of first things first. You and your body are number one. People may fault you for this and send criticisms your way, but they will understand later. Either way, we needn't internalize their insults. Dwelling on negativity is not beneficial to our health. What happens when you're in the hospital with a serious illness or injury? That's right. Someone else takes over your role. Our friends and relatives will not suffer for lack of attention. They are not being selfish either. They are just trying to secure their interests. Who can blame them? This is what being human is about. It's the nature of every creature to get its needs met.

What is the connection between "needs" and the functioning of our bodies? First, you should know that our bodies have definite needs of their own. Since our internal structures are alive, they have special needs too. This includes both physical and emotional needs. I proposed that the intelligent members of our bodies have feelings. Those uncountable personalities we know as the little minds are susceptible to the full range of emotions we generate including fear, love, anger, joy, and peace.

The truth is, your body needs you to "pay attention." What is attention? My definition of attention is **an act of consideration or courtesy, which demonstrates affection or love.** It also means **thoughtful consideration to the wants and needs of another to the exclusion of all else. Any sentient being is deserving of kindhearted attention.**

We should give priority to our bodies for this special treatment. What could be more valuable to us than the very thing that sustains our essence? Some of us decide to give preferential treatment to our vehicles over our bodies (not that cars aren't important).

We have an intimate relationship with our bodies and a mutual co-existence. We should realize that our bodies are companions to us. Every single cell possesses in our bodies knowledge of our most private thoughts. Our relationship with our bodies is markedly different from the human relationships we keep. For one, our bodies will not judge or criticize us. They will not develop any real hatred or resentment towards us. Though they may express certain basic emotions, such as anger (you may have heard of irritable bowel syndrome), they are not necessarily directed towards us. They may simply be expressing discontent or dissatisfaction.

Our bodies operate best from the experience of love, much as pets do. The little minds are motivated to please us. The trick is that they need to have that love returned. Our bodies like acknowledgement for their superior effort. They just ask for a little credit. They need the same kind of appreciation we give to other objects, plants, animals and people having special meaning to us. We tend to notice the importance of our insides only when we are sick.

In addition, our bodies expect first class treatment. They do not take kindly to being treated second best. Remember, they serve a vital role for us. I say this again because our good health is more valuable than all the gold in Fort Knox. It's surprising how some people will take enormous risks with their bodies. Eating 68 hot dogs in ten minutes in a contest does not sound healthy. Imbibing alcohol and illegal drugs is yet another activity your body will not tolerate. What would your body think about exposure to toxic chemicals without using the proper protection? I know someone who, out of youthful indiscretion, had the idea of putting LSD (acid) in his eyes to get a better trip. What he got was legally blind. These pursuits are unnecessary. Why would we do this to ourselves? I don't think anyone does these things with the intention of harming themselves. No one wants that. We just want to see how far we can push our bodies. It's okay to test your limits, but just be careful how you go about doing it. Now let's look at needs a little more closely.

Maslow's Pyramid

In his 1943 paper "A Theory of Human Motivation," Abraham Maslow created his famous "hierarchy of needs" pyramid. I can explain it this way:

Physiological

The bottom layer of this pyramid represents human physiological needs. This includes air, water, food, sex, and other factors related to homeostasis. This accounts for the basics, without which we would soon perish. It should be obvious that these needs are not negotiable. Common sense tells us this. These needs are the ones that come first. We will do whatever it takes to get the basics. What will you do to try to get air if it's difficult? How many of you can comfortably hold your breath more than a minute? What can we say about food and water? Are they a priority? What will the average person do to get these? Yes, it's true; sex is a basic need too. It's necessary to our well being, although some will debate this point. It's clear to me that our bodies need all of these basic items. It needs no clarification. So, let's move on.

Safety

The next rung up the ladder is safety. Safety gives us peace of mind. Let's look at the types of safety we need in our lives.

Personal safety: Personal protection is foremost in this band of the needs pyramid. That's why we sleep in houses. We require protection from the elements and intruders. We're able to sleep at night knowing our personal selves and belongings are safe from harm. Many crime victims develop serious mental illnesses due to a violation of safety. These unfortunate victims have had their space violated by another, and so their minds have constructed a defense against future attacks.

Financial security: Financial stability is a less-considered safety concern. People want to know that their money is safe from being stolen or depleted by circumstances that are outside of their control, such as job loss or prolonged illnesses. The average person feels at ease having enough money set aside to meet their future needs, while avoiding the paycheck-to-paycheck syndrome. Contrary to popular belief, most people like to keep their money in low-interest checking and savings accounts. This statement is especially true in a tough economy. Many people deal exclusively in cash. Their thinking is "better safe than sorry." Again, it allows them to sleep at night. Then there are those who risk their money in complicated investments that they do not fully understand. It's necessary to keep your head down when you're talking to a slick salesperson about his exotic investment deal. There are lots of swindlers in this world.

Job security: One's livelihood is another financial safety need that most people covet. People, who have worked in the same job for fifteen years and find themselves laid off due to an economic downturn often experience a high level of stress. They see their routines interrupted, and their financial means may be in question. Unemployment insurance isn't a very satisfying prospect. For the most part, people are happier when they have meaningful work to perform, as opposed to having nothing to do. A stable job with benefits is even better. A person cannot operate in limbo for long before it takes its toll.

Health-related safety: Is a health a priority? We're all concerned with our own well-being, even if we do not show it. In essence, we care about what happens to us, or at least we will care when we are in the emergency room. Most of us are terribly afraid of being hurt in any way. The state of our physical well-being is always somewhere in the back of our mind. We take any perceived threat against our persons seriously. We will quickly move to protect ourselves from the slightest sign of aggression. However, we do not want to be in such a position. We want nothing less than full respect for our safety and well-being. That's a reasonable expectation, isn't it?

Love

Let's talk about love. There are many kinds of love, including romantic, familial, friendship, communal, and divine love. One thing we seek to obtain from these loving relationships is acceptance and a sense of belonging. It is our innate desire to be wanted. That key motive leads to our two advanced needs for recognition and appreciation. They both fall under the umbrella of love.

Family: Many or most of us put family at the center of our lives. We are extremely tight with our families. We will go to any length to protect the members. This is especially true with our mothers and fathers. It's the first love we experience. There is no other love like it. It's a mighty bond. Our mothers and fathers brought us into this world, and we should thank them. They care for us, even if they do not show it. You may try to tell me different, but you can trust me, they do care. A mother, in particular, never loses her affection for her child. A mother and child have an uncommon bond that remains intact for life, even if one has passed on. It's inescapable. I'll bet some of you are saying "But my mother was horrible." This is just a tough exterior. They may seem mean at times (or all of the time), but there is another side that is not often seen. Feelings are not always apparent. It could be that your mother was discouraged from showing them, or perhaps some traumatic event may be the issue. Let me assure you, deep down the love is there. Even if the mother and the child connect for a few minutes, an eternal love is established. Just ask any woman who has experienced a miscarriage, or has put her baby up for adoption.

<u>Romantic</u>: In our intimate relationship(s), we see another powerful bond. I'm not talking about casual sex. That doesn't qualify as a romantic relationship. An intimate relationship is one in which we care more about our partner than we do for ourselves. This love comes from a place that is more spiritual in nature than the excitement we get from a brief romance or sexual encounter. Although it may start out with passion, our attraction to the other person doesn't depend on the surge of hormones and other chemicals to make the relationship flourish. Love might also form when both partners are willing to sacrifice all they have for each other. I know these statements are debatable and a little idealistic, but they work for our purposes. Self-sacrifice is a tricky subject. I'll tackle that in a bit.

Though not every intimate relationship lasts forever, they always remain with us. We will always have a strong connection to that special person. Somehow, the feelings we have will continue long after we have departed from this world. This is true even if we have decided we can't stand the person. We should be grateful for having this experience. Some people never get the chance.

The sacred bond that develops between two people is a powerful love that the body needs and absorbs into itself. If the super mind is contented, its employees will be happy, as well. Our bodies thrive on the personal attention we get from others, especially the kind that offers nurturing and affection. That closeness brings our bodies the security they require to function at their optimum.

Friends: Our friends encourage us in achieving our goals, and console us in our defeats. People say a true friend is always there for you. That sounds like a fair statement. If a friend isn't there for you, then he or she is certainly not someone you can count on, especially at crunch time. Therefore, we can say that friends support each other in both good and bad times.

Can anyone live without friendship? There are some hermits in this world, but even they require a certain amount of human contact to survive. We need each other. Though we may think we can do it all by ourselves, we quickly discover this isn't the case. We can accomplish much more in twos and threes than we can alone. As the saying goes, two heads are better than one, and I say that three heads are better than two are. Big things happen when people come together. I recall a statement made by US businessman and presidential candidate Ross Perot, when he was asked the secret to his success. Perot replied he surrounds himself with successful people. You will learn through your own research that this strategy has led to the success of our most admired leaders. Never underestimate the power of the mass mind. I will be discussing this collective giant later.

My position is that love should also be a basic need because humans cannot live without it. However, on this hierarchal pyramid, love is a higher need moving toward self-actualization. Fair enough. It is my personal belief that the Collective Consciousness dreamed the world into existence with nothing less than absolute love. Everything requires love. Nothing lives separately from it. The whole universe from its conception is nothing more than love. I assume that everyone has heard the saying "money makes the world go 'round." A better way of saying this is "love makes the world go 'round." Those deprived of love will wither and die. Think of a baby that grows up without love. Can you guess what will happen? Well, there is a strong possibility the baby will become dysfunctional in his or her adult life. Things like mental illness, addiction, debt, violence, and criminal behavior can set in. It's true that all of these terrible conditions will emerge from lack of affection.

Harlow Experiments: Some of you may recall from your high school and college psychology classes the famous monkey experiments conducted by Harry Harlow. The experiments involved separating a baby monkey from its mother and substituting her with a wire mother that would only feed it. Another group of monkeys was comforted with a cloth mother. After a while, researchers observed that the monkeys suffered from the developmental delays that included emotional and behavioral issues. Although I consider the experiments abusive, they clearly demonstrate the case for "maternal deprivation syndrome," which is separation from a mother figure. There are actual chemical changes that take place in the brain resulting from lack of touching and affection.[11, 12]

Romanian Orphans: Another investigation, conducted by Mary Carlson, associate professor of neuroscience and psychology at Harvard Medical School, looked at the orphans of the post-Nicolae Ceausescu Romanian regime. Under Ceausescu's harsh rule and drive for population growth, Romanian families found they were unable to care for their children, so they turned them over to orphanages that were grossly inadequate for taking on the parental role. It's estimated that there were over 150,000 children occupying these poorly managed orphanages. The childcare workers often had more than twenty infants to tend to at any given time. When scientists came to inspect the orphanages in 1989, they found children who had behaviors much like Harlow's monkeys. Some of the children displayed almost autistic–like mannerisms. Scientists observed the children to have severely delayed motor and cognitive functioning. Most interestingly (and sadly), their physical growth, was stunted. As the orphans progressed in age, they exhibited inappropriate social behavior. Many of these orphans ended up homeless. Still, other orphans, found themselves in unconventional occupations, suitable for their abnormal behaviors.[13]

Esteem

Coming in at a close second to self-actualization is self-esteem. Self-esteem is a cousin of self-respect. If you have self-respect, you most likely possess self-esteem. Self-respect has to do with the image we hold of ourselves. One definition for self-respect is showing honor to oneself. Alternatively, self-respect means holding oneself in high regard. One way we're guaranteed to lose our self-respect is to take on the views and opinions that others have of us. What does this mean? That's easy. Let's say you stay home from work one day because you have a cold. When you return to work the next day, your boss calls you lazy. If you agree with him, you lose your self-respect. If you take on the boss's negative view of yourself as being a lazy person, you will become lazy in a real way. This is what happens when we choose to adopt another's false opinion of us. It's not who we are. We know very well who we are, better than anyone else. Yet for some reason, we value everyone else's beliefs and opinions more than our own. It's a strange situation. Yet we all do it to some extent.

This may be because the opinions are coming from people we admire (or fear) like our parents, a teacher, a religious leader, a close friend, or some person we look up to. This scenario is loaded with emotion, as we have an enormous conflict when it comes to pleasing these folks and maintaining a reasonable amount of self-respect. Therapists earn their living helping people work through this issue.

Sometimes others don't agree with us (a little understatement). They unintentionally or perhaps deliberately try to run our lives because they think they know what is best for us. These are the little tyrants in our lives. I'd say most of these people are well intentioned. They are in our lives because they care. However, just because they do not agree with how we do things, does not mean we have to change for them. Having a sense of self-worth is akin to being true to ourselves. It means being who we are. It also means following our passion, and not letting the world dissuade us from following it. We have to remember that we're not at anyone's mercy. We are in charge of own thoughts and behavior. Our views and opinions are what matter to us, while still respecting those of others. We have to live with ourselves until we die… so get comfortable.

I'm going to digress for a moment and explore another reason for low self-esteem. Just stay with me on this. It's important. What happens is *we* (not someone else) *tell ourselves,* we're not worthy and then we find evidence to support it. You might say, "I'm a loser." Then you go about naming your apparent failures to justify this unproductive statement with negative remarks like, "I was bankrupt at 25, divorced at 35, and I'm now living with my parents." Why wouldn't you have low self-esteem with a personal outlook like that? I mean, it's not the ideal situation, but calling yourself names isn't helping. It's imperative we remember that these things are just events. They have no real meaning except the meaning we give to them. Divorce is just divorce. It's not good or bad. Society has given it a negative connotation. So what about it?

This is how to handle what others think of us and how to eliminate any self-loathing. Such destructive thoughts cannot have a hold on us unless we allow them. Learn to look at critical opinions, negative comments, and cynical remarks for what they are. They have no power. Take things in stride. Don't internalize such statements, especially when someone puts offensive language and unusually strong emotion into them. When we take on the opinions of others, we change the way we see the world and ourselves.

Here, is an example of this process. Most of us have seen the silly funhouse mirrors at amusement parks. Can you remember how these mirrors make your body appear distorted? One makes you look like a beanstalk, and the other makes you look like a plump dwarf. Is that how we look? It depends. If someone calls you fat, tubby, chunky, or some similar name, and you believe it, you will from that moment on, see yourself as the plump dwarf. It will become a reality for you. Without being a doctor, I would venture to say that this has something to do with how anorexia and bulimia work. This can also lead to an illness called body dysmorphic disorder (BDD). BDD is a serious medical condition in which the person suffering has a unhealthy obsession on certain parts of their body, such as the nose, weight, or hair. It's a distorted view of ourself.

In our society, we're preoccupied with being "perfect." We all know what the perfect body should look like. We see this image splashed on the cover of all of the magazines in the checkout line. They push it in our faces on television. Most of us have bought into it. We want to be like the "beautiful people." Therefore, we purchase all the diet pills and the exercise machines in an attempt to achieve that ideal figure. The weight loss industry takes in about 30 to 40 billion dollars a year. In actuality, all that they offer us is a distortion of reality and false hope. Their products do nothing more than to insult us. This makes us lose confidence in ourselves. When we do not achieve perfection, we assume that we have failed. After that, we proceed to beat ourselves up. That isn't necessary and only perpetuates the problem.

The perfection we're hoping for cannot be attained. Perfection is something you strive to reach. It's more of a timeless journey, than a final destination. It's like gymnastics. Gymnasts work all day and all night perfecting their routines, so they can win a competition. They need straight tens to get a perfect score. Most gymnasts will never get that far. And what if the gymnast does get that perfect score? Is that all there is? Does she exclaim: "Wow! That was great! Now I can retire." Of course, she doesn't. The gymnast starts training for the next competition.

Here's another example. There is a low-level employee working in a large corporation. He hates his menial job and dreams of being a senior manager. That's perfection to him. It does not get any better than that. So this low-level employee rises to the top and becomes a senior manager like he's always wanted. Guess what. He realizes it's not the top, and it's not perfect. What should we take away from this story? We should strive for perfection even though we will never get there. This is part of integrity. It's simply *doing the best you can*. Don't despise the process. Accept where you are and be ready to make improvements. Accepting your situation does not mean you are giving up or surrendering in any way. In this, case, acceptance means being okay with you and where you are in life. However, it doesn't mean staying where you are. Keep moving or fade away.

Be sure you don't put too much pressure on yourself. Perfection is a demanding proposition. Your body can't handle that kind of stress. Your body does need challenges, but you should always know your body's limits. Your body knows that perfection starts in the mind. The pursuit of perfection is necessary to test the human spirit. Your body is involved in this process. Personal growth is a consequence of the trials that you will inevitably face.

Some people think this world is not perfect because of all the terrible things that seem to happen every day. This creates a quandary because God is supposed to be perfect, and yet God birthed an imperfect world. How can that be? Let me explain. There is no imperfection; there is only change. Everything is growing, aging, and continually moving. That includes all animals, plants, minerals, and everything else that exists. This principle is absolute. Some things change so fast that we don't even see it happen. Other things may make a noticeable change over thousands of years. What about those objects, animals, civilizations, and ideas that have become extinct? That's called transformation. These things have simply taken on a new form. That is true evolution. I propose that change is perfection. I'll call this "perfection of the emerging consciousness" or just perfection of consciousness." Our godly source does not make mistakes. Spiritual evolution is part of the Infinite's master plan. Can you argue with the creator about how he or she (God is genderless) does his job? Okay then. Let's move on.

Deficiencies

Maslow referred to the bottom four layers of the pyramid as "deficiency needs," or "d-needs." The reason behind this arrangement should be getting clearer. As I discussed, in each of the middle three layers, deficiencies in the areas of safety, love, and self-esteem can cause severe psychological trauma. Most of the emotional illnesses people experience involve deficiencies in these areas. It's serious business. Not only must our needs be satisfied at these levels, but we must also conquer them. We cannot hope to move from the bottom to the top without mastering each level. If we cannot become 100% stable in our physiological needs, we will not be able to move to the level of safety. Nor can we claim self-actualization until we have mastered love.

Mastering a need takes place when we overcome all of the obstacles and circumstances that keep us from fully enjoying the benefits of that level. Mastering those needs means that you feel confident in your ability to succeed. You'll find that stress isn't such a significant factor in your life now. You are free from the nasties we call depression and anxiety. There is no longer a need for heavy doses of anti-depressants and addictive tranquilizers to keep us functioning.

In order to master a need, you must be determined to overcome any problem areas in your life. After making an intention, you must have the resolve to see it through. Your body places considerable importance on this commitment, since it shares in your victories. When the deficiencies are satisfied you will be faultless to a certain degree, and your body will celebrate. The little minds seek to enter into a harmonious relationship with the super mind. We all want to be right with the world. Just to emphasize, the phrase "little minds" does not mean lower minds or lesser minds. They are powerful beings just as we are.

As an investigator for so many years, I have come across plenty of decent people in complicated situations that would qualify as needy. This occurs in the areas of infidelity, child custody, child support collections, and criminal defense, to name a few. Many of these people are at their wits' end with their significant other (or perhaps not so significant in their eyes). They will say they have endured a lifetime of misery. They will do just about anything to get revenge for their mistreatment

Over fifteen years ago, a woman called me because her ex-husband was terrorizing her in a real way. As we talked, she stated that she would like to have her ex killed. I laughed this comment off and told the woman to call me back when she was interested in a real solution. Sometime later, it dawned on me that she might have been serious about the hitman idea. It's one of those feelings that come from years of psychic sleuthing (humorously). While I cannot get into the specifics of the case, let's just say that this situation was handled appropriately. My final thought on this is to ask the question, "Who in their right mind calls a private investigator out of the phone book to murder someone?" I'm certainly not interested in being the subject of a made-for-television drama.

Highly privileged people have the most difficulty mastering their needs. You'll hear them exclaim, "I can do whatever I want." That is a reckless attitude. Although these people like to put on a show of superiority, they are thoroughly entrenched in feelings of deficiency. I know that many people fantasize about putting a hit on their partner from time to time because of the extreme stress they are experiencing. Under these conditions, a person might say to his or her partner in a heated argument, "I wish you were dead." You can imagine where carrying out this thought out would get you. This attitude is certainly not in the realm of self-actualization. This low-level thinking leads to anger, regret, fear, resentment, bitterness, etc. These emotions keep us trapped in whatever level we're presently working in. We're certainly not in a race, but to keep our sanity we should be making progress.

Only a few of my cases were this extreme. However, the majority of my clients did, in fact, involve people who were not getting their needs met. It was heartbreaking to see this day in and day out. That is why I prefer working with people who are seeking to better themselves.

Deficiencies will poke holes in your energy reserves leaving you depleted. When you clear out space inhabited by beneficial entities, leaving it empty, you make room for harmful invaders to move in.

These intruders bring disease and contamination with them. Remember, wherever there is a need, there will be something ready to fill it. Predators of all kinds exist because there is a need or a void present. I'm using the word predator in a general sense. If we are not careful, harmful invaders, such as parasites will make their home in empty spaces within our bodies.

In general, when people are desperate, they fall victim to predators. To illustrate how one can be taken advantage of by a predator, I'd like to offer this little piece. The other day a person I know well, who likes to participate in clinical research studies, came to me for advice concerning a private study he found on Craigslist. The ad stated that the participants would use their natural weight loss product for 60 days while monitoring their weight at home, and receive a total payment of $1,500.00 upon completion. My friend responded with interest by email. Their reply directed him to fill out a short questionnaire on their website. Sure enough, he received an immediate response approving him as a study participant. The questionnaire then instructed him to visit another web page to order the "free" product. Not surprisingly, the site required him to pay for the shipping charges. This is where the story ends. You should never pay any money to volunteer for a research study. You are the one being paid.

Complementary and alternative medicine (CAM) accounts for a hefty chunk of the consumer market. One estimate for 2003 puts consumer spending on CAM services and dietary supplements at $54 billion. I'd like to point out, that out of this figure; $34 billion was spent on services such as chiropractic and massage therapy.[14]

Based on this information, we can say that most people have a strong will to live and a desire to maintain their health. We eat healthy, exercise (if we can), and take medication or whatever treatments are available. Often this isn't enough. Many of us look to alternative medicine for a boost. Some work quite well. Others are scams. These scams are all over the Internet – different concoctions said to make us feel better. Companies make claims that their natural substances aid the body in certain ways to alleviate their problems. These fraudsters promise the world, but deliver little, or nothing. In addition, the questionable products sold by these companies rarely measure up to the standards of those requiring federal approval. Their products don't have to meet the stringent standards set forth by the government, because their ingredients and intended use, do not meet the FDA's definitions. I am always an advocate for safety.

These peddlers of false hope exploit the consumer's belief that their products are safe because they are "natural." This reassuring word seems to justify the unseen risks. We all want to feel better, but we need to find safe alternatives. If your physicians have told you that you are terminally ill, and you know it to be true, then you should take whatever steps you feel will return you to a healthy state. If you are trying to lose a few pounds, however, please do not spend thousands of dollars on products that have a zero return on investment. We need to be informed. We cannot allow ourselves to come under the spell of these charlatans. Don't assume a product is safe, just because a person or company says it's natural. Look into it.

The tools of the Body Alive Principle use creative visualization and affirmative language to manage the body. These established techniques safely facilitate the healing process. I don't suggest this will be a surefire cure for any particular medical condition. It may be a miracle cure for some people and perhaps a level of relief for others. The modalities of the Body Alive Principle have clearly demonstrated their value in the healing arts. The physicians of the great civilizations of the past have successfully employed these and other mental techniques for healing. The choice is yours as to whether or not you accept the Body Alive Principle as a qualified alternative therapy.

You will find other high quality publications, which deal exclusively with visualizations and affirmations. I recommend *Creative Visualization* by Shakti Gawain. It's an excellent choice for further reading. This book has sold over three million copies to date. It has been well received by alternative health practitioners and people from all walks of life.

Self-actualization

Self-actualization is at the top of the pyramid. This position denotes our highest need. This comes after all needs at the bottom are satisfied. What is self-actualization? It sounds like an enigmatic concept. Self-actualization is essentially the aim of reaching one's full potential.

Self-actualized people have a heightened awareness of their environment. They have a silent knowing. Self-actualizers can perceive those things that are beyond what others comprehend. This experience is more like a heightened human experience than a mystical event. It's a bit non-ordinary in the sense that most people are not self-actualized. It's something of a rarity in industrialized societies when compared to the large population in these countries. The good news is that most self-actualizers are not celebrities and anyone with determination can reach this exceptional state.

Self-actualization is a process. It follows a path of personal growth and development. It's the daring process of finding oneself. It starts with the "Who am I?" question, followed by "What is my purpose?" There are many questions directed at oneself in the beginning. Such questions are nothing less than an expression of defiance to our controlling ego. The process of becoming self-actualized destroys the ego. Therefore, expect resistance. An oppressive regime never surrenders its power without a fight. It isn't an easy path to tread in the beginning.

Self-actualized people show personal qualities and habits that are markedly different that of the non-actualized. Some historical figures that Maslow would have considered self-actualizers include:

- Thomas Jefferson
- Martin Luther King, Jr.
- Albert Einstein
- Jane Addams
- Eleanor Roosevelt

The Traits of a Self-Actualized Individual

1. They are realistic.

Self-actualized people perceive reality clearly and accurately. Practice seeing things for the way they are, rather than how you think they are. There is a vast difference between the two. Leave your judgmental thoughts and colored emotions out of it. I have to say that being a detective for over 18 years has helped give me clarity. You should always seek the truth in all cases. The truth is subject to individual interpretation, so be objective. Developing this habit will serve you well in all your pursuits.

You should also be logical and efficient. You want to keep your head about you. Don't give in to vagueness and uncertainty – work with them. Your goal isn't to shut ambiguity out of your life, since the world is full of it. Ambiguity is your friend; it brings spice to life. Your logical sense will transform ambiguity, if you insist on doing things the right way. Be aware that logic is not your only tool. Relying solely on reason to get through a complicated situation is a mistake. You will know the right way of doing things when you have started on this path. You are seeking clarity, and the process of self-actualization makes that inevitable.

2. They do not fear the unknown.

- The unknown represents the things that are normally beyond our reach. This hidden knowledge is inaccessible through the usual channels. The phrase "thinking outside the box" originated here.

- We draw inspiration from the unknown. It holds promise for the thinkers and hope for the dreamers.

- It spurs our imagination. On the one hand, we fear it, and on the other, it intrigues us. We are like a puppy venturing out into the world for the first time.

- The unknown instills faith in us that there exists something greater than ourselves.

- It brings out the best in the human experience.

3. They exercise acceptance.

My definition of acceptance calls for one to allow both physical and nonphysical things to be just as they are in whatever state they exist. I am talking about acceptance in the universal sense. This includes acceptance of yourself, as well as acceptance of things outside of yourself, and outside of your control. When you are able to accept who you are, you are then able to accept your circumstances and those of the world at large. Acceptance is nebulous and covers a lot of territory. It's difficult to pin down in a few sentences. From my perspective, acceptance means, "it is what it is." That means not putting any labels or judgments on the person, object, or event we are observing. A person or object will always stand on its own whether we approve of it or not. The entity's existence does not depend on whether we believe in it.

It's true that a self-actualized person has lost his self-importance. Self-actualized people do not need to prove anything to anyone. Self-actualizers know themselves. They are confident about their lifestyle choices. They are not burdened by public opinion, although they are mindful of the thoughts of others. Self-actualizers realize that their circumstances are only temporary, and are subject to change. There is a difference between accepting something with a feeling of helplessness, and accepting a thing to show honor to it, while having the courage to improve on it. Our relationship with our bodies should reflect the latter.

The body has a need for us to accept our respective situations and make whatever improvements are necessary for us to function at an optimum level. The qualifier to this statement is "when necessary." Too often, we can't leave well enough alone. This has to do with the misuse of perfection.

Remember the famous serenity prayer by Reinhold Niebuhr:

> God grant me the serenity
> to accept the things I cannot change;

courage to change the things I can;
and wisdom to know the difference.

Society has trained us to be unhappy with whatever we have, especially our bodies. Every advertisement sings out "You are not good enough!" Hundreds of unhealthy advertising images bombard unsuspecting consumers every day. If you turn on your television for an hour at any time of the day to virtually any channel, you will see several commercials telling you that your body is imperfect. You will be delighted to see commercials for make-up, shampoo, sexy clothes, and weight loss contraptions. I feel this is highly offensive to our intelligence. And strangely enough, a lot of these commercials seem to air in conjunction with the soap operas.

The next issue I will discuss is that, if you do not like your body, you are doing yourself a great disservice. The body responds to these messages in a negative way. We subject ourselves to self-loathing for many reasons. Let's examine the reasons behind how we got to this point. Our well-intentioned parents taught us to be humble, reserved, modest, and soft-spoken. They taught us to limit our self-expression and ask for nothing. We developed a sense of powerlessness. We felt inadequate. Some of us carried this sense of helplessness throughout life. Soon we identified with it. It became who we are. As a result, our bodies suffered. Our bodies became a reflection of what we thought of ourselves. We stopped taking care of our bodies. We ate terrible foods. We took to indulging in fatty, greasy junk food. We decided to take the easy way out and stop at our favorite fast food restaurant on the way home from work.

Exercise was unthinkable because we were too sick and tired. I wonder why? We didn't go to the doctor for our routine checkups. Our sleep was compromised because we were up all night doing work for the next day, or we just couldn't sleep from worry. Naps were a joke, and relaxation was the time spent waiting at a red light. Please don't feel guilty or ashamed if you identify with this profile. I've done this myself in recent times. My point is, many of us have seriously neglected our bodies for years. As you can see, it takes a while to get into a pattern like this, and it will take some time to get out. Before going on a diet, or attempting to lose weight, accept your body just the way it is. Be okay with yourself. Genuinely accepting yourself will make your weight loss efforts much more successful.

4. They are private.

A self-actualized person knows the importance of privacy. Society uses the term "private" to describe these people. When used in this context, private is considered a term of respect. Someone may have said to you, "I respect your privacy." Then there are those people who find private individuals to be mysterious. Still others believe a private person has something to hide. Carlos Castaneda is the author of *The Teachings of Don Juan: A Yaqui Way of Knowledge* and several other books dealing with shamanism. During his lifetime, Castaneda was almost invisible to the world. He gave few interviews and did not allow journalists to take his photograph. Privacy was part of the philosophy taught to Castaneda by his teacher Don Juan.

Privacy can also be associated with solitude. People often seek privacy because of an innate desire to be alone. Perhaps they seek solitude to experience inner peace. Some problem-solvers have a deep desire to get away from the world and be with themselves. They may not even realize that this is the case.

This leads us to the misunderstood word "seclusion". In this case, seclusion means voluntarily and temporarily removing oneself from society to do inner work. There is a difference between physical and mental seclusion. Mental seclusion does not necessarily require physical seclusion. Many times people want physical seclusion to avoid distractions. Solitude is a fundamental characteristic of any meditation practice. Self-actualized people seek enlightenment through seclusion and meditation. Being alone with your greater self can be life changing. Any spiritual journey requires alone time to contemplate one's place in life.

Privacy also stems from the desire to stay out of the limelight and "keep a low profile." I refer you back to Castaneda. Self-actualized people have no need to brag or sing their own praises. They are confident in themselves and their abilities. They know who they are and what they are capable of accomplishing. Self-actualized people have already mastered the need for self-esteem. Privacy, not secrecy, has become a way of life for them.

5. They are problem-centered.

This person is by no means self-centered or egotistical. In fact, he or she is dedicated to improving the lives of others. I am describing a person who is deserving of the title of problem-solver. The problem-solver treats life's quandaries as situations in need of a solution. The list below identifies and explores the personal traits possessed by an exceptional problem-solver in detail. This section also looks at how these characteristics apply to the mind-body connection and the Body Alive Principle:

The Nine Qualities of an Exceptional Problem-Solver

A. They are Determined to Succeed.

Those with an unwavering mindset are able to take lemons and turn them into lemonade. Determined problem-solvers find a way to make existing conditions work both efficiently and effectively. They do not yield to conventional limitations. Problem-solvers can overcome any obstacle. They will go over them, under them, around them, or plow straight through them if necessary. Problem-solvers will work to find the answer(s). Problem-solvers can be persistent. They do not give up easily. With a can-doer, anything is possible. One of my favorite maxims is "There's a way to do everything."

A can-do attitude will get you through the hard times. What's that saying? "When the going gets tough, the tough get going." There's a reason why these sayings have longevity. They have wisdom. You've got to forge ahead in spite of opposition. If Abraham Lincoln had listened to his critics and bowed to his early defeats, he would never have become our 16th president.

Our bodies share in the excitement of this "go-getter" attitude. The super mind sets high standards and then the little minds work at achieving them. Personal motivation is beneficial to our bodies. In effect, the little minds become equally excited. They will generate their own fire, which in turn will provide you with your get-up-and-go. It's surprising how much energy this mentality will generate. This high energy brings a sense of exhilaration to your body. Everything seems to come alive.

Problem solving is the essence of investigative work. If you are interested in developing your problem-solving skills in a radical way, you might get an internship at your local detective agency. It will teach you life lessons that you cannot get anywhere else.

B. They Think Outside the Box

A person who defaults to redefining a problem is a classic problem-solver. This practice involves looking at things from a different perspective. The problem-solver is trying to understand the situation and find a new angle from which to tackle it. When considering a new blueprint to work from, the problem-solver leaves all options on the table and examines them carefully, looking for the right fit. There is a definite answer for each of life's mysteries. Sometimes the answer is right in front of our nose, and sometimes it isn't so obvious; it takes our creative energies to make those answers visible. Our creativity is usually the best tool for securing a meaningful answer. It's also the one we tend to consider last – not consciously; it's just that we forget it's there.

Our bodies engage themselves in redefining our problems. The body is extraordinarily proficient at finding ways to cure itself of illnesses, for example. It looks at ways for adapting to adversity. If you experience a traumatic event, your body will develop complex coping mechanisms to deal with it. Our bodies are intelligent and creative; the little minds are able to act as a team of medical investigators joining forces to resolve health issues.

C. They create highly effective systems.

Successful people use systems. Establishing a system indicates intent. Intention leads to achievement of purpose. An effective system means the difference between ultimate success and outright failure (in human terms). A well-designed system does many things including saving time, energy, and money. The key is to find a system that works. It does little good to keep doing the same thing repeatedly without satisfaction. If that is the case, you might as well take the day off and go golfing. Identifying a system that works can be a daunting task. Once a personal system has been found, many people will spend a lifetime trying to perfect its finer points. That's okay. When you have an unbeatable system in place, it's like finding the proverbial yellow brick road.

One way to cut down on the work involved in developing a system is to borrow one from someone who is already successful (this is not to say that innovation can't grow out of this method). The name of this practice is "modeling". If you are an aspiring actor, you might model an actor who has already hit the big-time. It's unlikely that a stranger is going to give you their personal success system, however. A problem-solver will still be able to get that information. Uncovering secrets is the nature of problem-solvers. It's what makes a problem-solver worth his or her weight in gold.

Let's look at some wildly successful businesses, like McDonald's, Burger King, and Dunkin' Donuts (I have no great preference any of these). How did these powerhouse corporations become so successful? That's right! They developed a system. What is their system? I don't know, but if you could figure it out, and put it to use, you might become a multimillionaire. There is one unmistakable commonality among these giants. It's rather obvious. They are all franchises. Franchises are able to reproduce the success of their first business to form new businesses. It's like the process of cell division, or mitosis. The original business continues splitting and making exact replicas of itself.

Systems are not one size fits all. A problem-solver realizes there is just one system that will lead him to the golden prize. It's not just finding a system that's important. It's necessary to find one that works for you. This seems like an oversimplified statement. Nonetheless, it's a truly powerful message.

Of course, our bodies have their own systems. In fact, our bodies are the authority on systems. Our bodies have created incredibly successful systems for your benefit. We would not have a body without these systems. Here, they are, just for reference:

- Circulatory
- Digestive
- Endocrine
- Immune
- Lymphatic
- Muscular
- Nervous
- Reproductive
- Respiratory
- Skeletal
- Urinary

These body systems are mission critical. If something goes wrong with any of them, you will certainly know it. Give the little minds some credit for doing their jobs so well, even if they compromised. In fact, give them even more praise if you have a disability. They like that a lot. As I have tried to impress upon you, these systems receive our mental and emotional signals – that is a key point. Please give credit where credit is due.

D. They avoid relying solely on experience.

Experience is of immense help in navigating this complex world. There is no substitute for hard-earned experience. However, over-reliance on what we know can lead us into a ditch. Experience has its limitations. If you over-rely on what you know, you will soon discover that you know very little. There are too many variables in life to assume that you have the right answers based on what your experience has taught you. Like the stock market, past performance is no guarantee of future profits. It isn't reasonable to assume that an experience you had in the past will have the same results in a similar situation today. You will be severely disappointed when your project has an outcome that is different from what you had planned.

Successful problem-solvers have learned to rely on their intuitive sense as opposed to their experience in resolving a predicament. Use experience as a guideline to get you headed in the right direction. Do not draw conclusions using only experience. Experience creates a frame for the house you are building. If you have enough time, you might try contemplating the issue you are working on. Problem-solvers realize experience becomes incredibly powerful when augmented with other internal means. Creativity is one of those tools. Use creativity to discover new ways of approaching the issue. Creativity is your friend. It will take you down unexplored avenues like a mouse to the cheese.

Try looking at the situation from the standpoint of an outside observer. Use your imagination. Most importantly, you should avoid making hasty decisions based on your experience. In time, this will lead to trouble. Instead, use your intuition. I will be talking about this highly useful tool shortly.

An intuition versus experience scenario presents itself when we look at how a mouse in a labyrinth will try a different path after going down a dead-end. Humans, on the other hand, will keep going down that same dead end street time after time hoping to reach the prize. As an investigator, I found people to be predictable. This fact made doing my job much easier. People like their routines and rituals. They are uncomfortable trying something new. It's been said we are creatures of habit. That being the case, I think this is an excellent time to bring up the pothole story. I think it fits in well with this section.

The Pothole Story: A Tale of Victory

One day a man was walking down a street. He unexpectedly fell into a wide pothole that was obstructing his path. He was able to climb out of this pothole with great difficulty, and with the help of strangers who had witnessed his misfortune.

The next day the man took the same route down the same street and fell into the same deep pothole. Just as before, he climbed out with the assistance of sympathetic strangers. This time he did it with less difficulty.

On the third day, the man proceeded down the same street just as he had the day before. This time he saw the pothole, but he fell into it again. He learned how to get out of the pothole from the previous falls. So, the man dusted himself off and with some difficulty climbed out of the pothole without assistance.

On the fourth day, the man saw the pothole and attempted to go around it. He fell into the pothole once more, but was able to climb out with great ease.

On the fifth day, the man clearly saw the pothole. With some effort, he managed to maneuver around it and went on his way.

On the following day, the man saw the pothole obstructing his way and decided to take a safer route. The man continued on to his destination with a sense of victory at having overcome his challenge.

There are several variations of this story floating around the Internet. This story certainly gives a little insight into the human condition. There are probably several lessons evident in this story. To me, it's a good analogy of how we as humans, are stuck in our ways, and fail to see the pitfalls that are keeping us from our success. It takes a long time for us to recognize that we are our own worst enemy. In many ways, we sabotage ourselves and deny ourselves victory. It's too bad we must learn our life lessons this way. Interestingly, I've found it's far easier for us to solve other people's problems than to deal with our own. Life can be a challenge, and that's a good thing. Just don't get too caught up in it.

E. They appreciate the value of conflict.

It seems there is always resistance when seeking a solution to a problem. People tend to disagree either in part or entirely. Each person believes he or she is right. This is a fundamental concept. The need to be right seems to be an innate and almost natural disposition for most of us. Being right is a way of feeding our ego. The self-righteous have a strong desire to have others adopt their views. There are a large number of privileged people in this country who insist others do things their way. It even became a famous slogan for Burger King, "Have it your way." Not that Burger King had any more of a hand in creating this condition than anyone else did. It borders on absurdity. There are even people who are willing to die to prove their beliefs are right. Of course, there are many motivations behind such acts. A lot of this has to do with how our parents or guardians raised us. I'm not trying to pick on parents, since we are all responsible for ourselves when we become adults.

Beware of self-righteous people who seek to block your forward progress. Problem-solvers will welcome such commotion as a way of bringing out the truth. Resistance encourages problem-solvers to forge ahead with enthusiasm. It invigorates them.

Problem-solvers need to have strong conflict management skills to make their way through the troubled waters created by mischief-makers. Problem-solvers will work with the self-righteous attitudes of other people to get their job done. A worthy problem-solver uses opposition to his or her advantage. Conflict is a way of generating new ideas that can lead to a solution. It's useful to look at conflict as an opportunity rather than an obstacle.

The body is equipped to transform conflict into something positive. Conflict is taking place in your body at this moment. Harmful bacteria and viruses continually test the body's defenses. Psychological pressure is another stress we inflict on our bodies. We also abuse our wonderful companions by consuming excessive amounts of junk food and harmful substances. If the stress the body experiences is not overwhelming, it will put up various forms of protection to deal with the assaults. This activity will efficiently remove harmful invaders and produce antibodies.

When microscopic invaders first attempt to enter the body, they encounter physical barriers like the skin and the internal linings of the airway and intestines. These barriers produce chemicals that prevent the spread of any unwelcome visitors. The release of acid in the stomach is an example of this.

The immune system uses white blood cells, or leukocytes, to identify and destroy invaders. The white blood cells are the sentinels of the body. They stand ready to repel any attack. They also produce antibodies that counteract the activities of pathogens. There are two types of leukocytes. The first are lymphocytes. These white blood cells allow the body to recognize and remember harmful invaders. Then there is *phagocytosis, a process in* which phagocytes swallow up intruders, using interferon enzymes to destroy them.

Our bodies know that conflict is a universal constant, like the struggle between dark and light. One is always trying to dominate the other. In fact, the physical universe itself is in a constant state of conflict. You may have heard the phrase "survival of the fittest." This phrase describes the incredible conflict that rages on in the universe. The body, with its own relentless internal warfare, strives to become stronger in the process. I believe the adage, "what doesn't kill you makes you stronger" is relevant to this discussion. My own theory is that the conflict in the body (and generally in life) has an unnamed benefit. I know I'm not the first to suggest this idea. For the sake of this book, I'll call it "constructive conflict dynamics." Conflict has a way of keeping the body on its toes and ready for anything. This is a beneficial state to be in, so long as it is not overwhelming. Though this may be a controversial idea, I'm confident in stating that stress may improve our lives. I believe our bodies view conflict or stress as a growth opportunity. Stress is indicative of change. The body needs change to grow. If the body overcomes a stressful event, it will become more resilient, and able to resist even the most severe attacks. Therefore, stress itself can be essential to our physical development. Stress presents a challenge. It is something we need to overcome (though not in all cases) in order to move up Maslow's pyramid.

Our bodies require both physical and spiritual growth. If you have accepted my theories up to this point, you might agree that our bodies need a connection to the creator. They have a yearning to feel one with the universe. Therefore, you could say that conflict brings about harmony between the mind, body, and spirit. Though I cannot say I've performed extensive research to prove this theory, I am personally inclined to believe that exposure to moderate stress improves our quality of life and that of our body.

F. They have a keen intuitive sense.

Intuition plays a vital role in the life of the problem-solver. Intuition also happens to be one of my favorite topics. Intuition is the immediate apprehension of knowledge without the use of reasoning processes. A problem-solver knows the answers often lie outside of the confines of linear thinking and does not rely on his or her experience alone. A problem-solver knows that there is another form of consciousness accessible to those with the requisite knowledge. It's exciting to know that this resource is available to anyone who seeks it. Not only can detectives use it, but each one of us possessing natural insight.

What is the source of this mysterious insight? No one living honestly knows. I believe it comes from the Universal or Collective Consciousness that is composed of the minds of every atom and structure that exists. This includes gases, light, and even thought. Some call this collective entity God. Some people describe God as a type of vibratory energy. This comes under the law of vibration, which asserts that all things exist in a vibratory state. However, the law of vibration is not the focus of this book. Numerous books and articles have given their attention to this fundamental principle. I do want to point out that the vibration theory is associated with the law of attraction. Many of you are probably familiar with this law. It is a fad these days. Just know that the law of attraction is only the tip of the iceberg. I can tell you there is much left to discover.

The Infinite Mind records each experience that manifests in the physical universe, almost like a video camera. This is true of all things. Events documented, would include, things like a wind blowing in a tree in merry old England in the 1400s. Every atom in the universe has equal access to this data. It is my unscientific opinion that each atom has all of the information ever known since the dawn of time. It's a lot like a gene, which contains the blueprints needed to replicate. I spoke of this earlier when I discussed the subject of cellular memory. This concept, the "Infinite Archive," also involves an adjoining principle that each one of us has complete access to this resource.

The popular term for this resource is "akashic records" or "book of life." Psychic Edgar Cayce popularized the idea of the Akashic records in the 1900s. Michael Newton, a hypnotherapist, explored this idea in his books *Journey of Souls and Destiny of Souls* and *Evidence of Life between Lives*. In the early 1900s, C.W. Leadbeater, noted for his metaphysical writings, also conducted research into the Akashic records.

The Infinite Archive is not the ultimate source of power. Humans get some funny ideas about twisting the nature of benign energies to suit their needs. The Infinite Archive is the ultimate repository of information, and yet, is more than just information contained in a massive hard drive. This Source is accessible anywhere and everywhere, past and future. The American government took a stab at using this resource for spying, by attempting to exploit what they called *remote viewing* (clairvoyance). Joseph McGoneagle, a former remote viewer for the US Army Intelligence, authored a book entitled *The Stargate Chronicles: Memoirs of a Psychic Spy* in which he shares his experience with Project Stargate. There is information about this research project all over the Internet. Some of this information is reliable, and much of it probably isn't. That's the nature of the endless Internet. My best advice is to look around and use your keen judgment to find credible sources. Just don't get caught up in the conspiracy theories.

In your meditation practice, you might find that the past and future do not seem to exist. That is the peculiar nature of time. When you finally understand time, you will realize that, in truth, we only exist in the present moment. There is only now. Time is simply a measurement between events. This will be a revelation for those of you who have not already discovered this supreme truth. For more information, please see *Journey of Souls: Case Studies of Life between Lives* and *Destiny of Souls: New Case Studies of Life between Lives*, both by Michael Newton.

The records can be retrieved in many ways, including through music, prayer, meditation, dancing, dreams, and visions. There are talented "psychics" who are able to achieve a higher level of success than the rest of us. On that note, I feel it's appropriate to bring up "sensitives".

Sensitives are the kind people who are highly receptive to the attitudes, feelings, and mental state of others. The feelings of these people may be easily hurt. They may also be quick to take offense and may be easily irritated. Some call a person with this quality "touchy." However, being highly receptive to the emotions of others, does not automatically qualify a person as "sensitive". The little minds must handle and transmit stimuli to the super mind in a particular way to make this talent possible.

Problem-solvers may be sensitive to impressions radiated by people and objects. Many problem-solvers do not even realize they possess this amazing ability. Just remember, you may not have been born with extra sensory skills, but you can develop them. And no one is denied access to these tools or the Infinite Archive. The Universal Intelligence always obeys equal opportunity laws.

How does intuition help the problem-solver? Intuition allows the person possessing this heightened ability to immediately, and directly perceive the answer to a problem through inspiration, revelation, or gifted insight. When this happens, one might say, "It came like a bolt from out of the blue." It's as if the answer suddenly appears in your mind. This can be an enormous relief after you've spent hours or even days laboring over an issue combing through every detail in vain. Sometimes we have to stop thinking so hard. Human thinking is limited. It uses reasoning to get the answers. Common sense, logic, and measurements govern the physical realm. More often than not, the answers lie outside these confines.

One way to gain unrestricted access to this powerful resource is to stop trying to control everything. You might recall the saying "Let go and let God." This is true regardless of what formalized religion you might follow. We would all do well to realize that we can't control anything outside of ourselves. It's been written by many authors that the best we can do is give a controlled response to what life throws at us. We can answer a matter presented to us in one of two ways. We either respond calmly and positively to a situation or react fiercely to it. A reaction is typically just a "knee-jerk reaction" to a startling or distressing event. Reaction comes from our primal instinct. A response is "controlled and planned." A certain amount of planning takes place before addressing the issue in front of us. If necessary, this reflective process can take place in a matter of seconds. A planned response clearly lends itself to a higher thought process. That's not to say that reaction is useless to us. Reaction serves a critical role in urgent situations.

One way to take a responsive position in life is to stop taking responsibility for the actions of others. This is our control instinct. You can only control *how you deal* with a given situation. You cannot control what others do or do to you. If you write an award-winning report at work and your boss says its garbage, that's not something you can control. You can't control what he says about it. You could rewrite that report a thousand times. Chances are your boss still won't accept it. Why? It's his disposition (I know some of you want me to say it's because he's a jerk). Everyone knows someone who can't be pleased. How should you respond to a person like this? That's easy. Don't take offense from his criticisms. Not responding is a response. Now maybe it's not so easy at first. Like everything else, you need to practice. Take a deep breath, collect your thoughts, and then respond. Eventually you'll be able to sort out what you are responsible for and what other people need to account for.

Responding to an event leaves our emotions out of the matter, leaving us with a clear mental state. Our emotions, as a problems-solving tool, will come into play in other acute situations. Sometimes being clear-headed is enough. Through regular practice, this open-mindedness enables us to receive cosmic guidance. This is the intuition of which I've been speaking. The bottom line is, when we change what we do on the inside, it has an equal effect on those things outside of us.

As a reminder, the body relates to conflict in much the same way we do. Since the body needs to be tested, it will welcome any challenge confident in its ability to overcome it. Our bodies will turn conflict and opposition into a positive encounter. This scenario works if we, the superior mind, are leading the way. The body can only put up a limited defense to confrontation. We are the ones who must take charge of the situation. Ultimately, the ability to overcome adversity lies with the superior mind. The body working under our leadership will become healthy and strong. You will know this is true because you will feel vibrant and alive. This is how the body shows its power.

An example of response versus reaction is maintaining a steady meditation practice, as opposed to taking prescription medication. Meditation is a proactive response whereas medication is reactive. A meditative response is putting up a defense against anything seen or unseen that may be a threat.

Meditation is one of the primary methods used for facilitating an empathetic connection with the body. In short, it's an excellent way to get in touch with the body. Meditation calms the mind and allows a spiritual connection to take place. There is an abundance of documented evidence available to substantiate the healing quality of meditation   Studies have shown that meditation is beneficial for the following:

- Reducing anxiety
- Lowering high blood pressure
- Lowering bad cholesterol
- Helping curb substance abuse tendencies
- Increasing intelligence (in the broad sense)
- Eliminating incidents of post-traumatic stress disorder (PTSD)
- Reducing cortisol

In meditation, you focus on a thought or feeling (at least that is how I have done it). In doing this, you turn your attention inwards. Your mind will try to escape this process. It will wander off into dreams and fantasies. Your job is to gently, bring your attention back. You shouldn't look at this as a power struggle, however. It's just part of the experience. You are not doing it wrong. There is nothing wrong with you.

There are many variations of meditation. Most popular meditation practices come from India, China, and Japan. A practice called mindfulness meditation is the one I have found most useful in implementing the Body Alive Principle. Mindfulness involves the conscious direction of one's awareness on certain parts of the body. A mindfulness practitioner undertakes each meditative session with intention. If you are being mindful, then you are paying attention. Your mind will wander off if given the opportunity. When this happens, you will need to return your focus back to the intention of your meditation. That is mindfulness as I experienced it. Obviously, this isn't always the case with other forms of meditation.

A consistent mindfulness practice is excellent for training yourself to focus on one task to the exclusion of all else. These tasks can include things such as eating and brushing your teeth. The idea is to experience the activity using all of your five senses. If you were brushing your teeth, you might notice the taste of the toothpaste, the feel of the bristles against your teeth, the sound the toothbrush makes, etc. You will become thoroughly engrossed in the experience. At some point, you might notice that you have shut out all other activity around you. This experiment shows the true power of the mind. There are some applications for pain management here. Being present with the pain is a significant step toward healing your mind and body. "Feeling the pain" has potential benefits. This is in contrast to "feeling no pain", which is essentially a state of numbness, usually chemically induced. Just remember, you do not want to ignore any pain. This exercise is about awareness. If meditation is too frustrating, then try this surefire pain elimination technique. The next time you feel achy and fatigued from your daily routines, drop a large rock on your foot; in a matter of seconds, your general discomfort will miraculously vanish. Try the meditation exercise first. You'll save yourself a hospital visit.

Mindfulness meditation involves becoming aware of what is going on inside of you as well as outside. A mindfulness "body scan" entails feeling out each part of your body and focusing on whatever sensations are noticeable. These sensations are typically physical, although you may get other feelings while doing this. This unique practice is exploratory and often leads to personal insights. You might find it unnerving to be with yourself at first. You will become aware of emotions and memories that are below the surface. It is to your advantage to deal with these experiences. It can be incredibly freeing.

Many consider John Kabat-Zinn Ph.D the central figure in the mindfulness movement. He is the founder of the Center for Mindfulness in Medicine, Health Care, and Society, at the University of Massachusetts Medical School. He has written a number of books on the subject. He also started the **Stress Reduction Clinic at the UMass** Medical School, which teaches mindfulness-based stress reduction (MBSR). I attended this program and found it to be well worth the investment.

Here, is a mindfulness meditation exercise you can try that is almost effortless if you are well enough to do it. It's best done lying down on a mat or a cushioned surface. Try to do it at a time that you will not be disturbed. Don't be discouraged if you are unable to complete it the first few times. Mindfulness is a practice that goes beyond any eight-week workshop.

Become aware of your body.
You might move your awareness down to your toes.
Notice any sensations in the toes.
Are they comfortable?
Do you feel any tingling or itching?
Are they warm or cold?

Don't be concerned as to whether you are doing it right.

Spend as much time as you need exploring this area.

Continue up your body this way.

Next, bring your awareness to your feet

Scan both feet for sensations.

Maybe you can feel the pressure of the soles of your feet against the floor.

Now move your awareness to your lower legs.

You will likely find your mind wandering. Thoughts will come and go. This is perfectly normal. Be aware of them. If these thoughts are not the subject of your meditation, just allow them to pass through. Then continue with your session.

Become aware of sensations where you are sitting or lying.

Wherever your body is positioned is fine. You may become aware of the surface your body is touching.

Moving up to your abdomen, you may notice sensations both outside and inside.

Explore what is happening inside your stomach.

Now move your awareness to your chest and lungs.

You might feel a sense of warmth or coolness present.

Note the rise and fall produced by your breathing.

You may also be aware of your heart beating.

Now go down to your fingers.

What do they feel like?

Do you notice any space between them?

Any stiffness?

Any other sensations?

Check your forearms.

Maybe you feel the pressure of your forearms against the surface on which you are sitting or lying.

Now move on to your upper arms.

What do you feel?

If you feel nothing, that is perfectly fine.

Scan your neck for anything that might be present.

Some people notice tension or tightness.

If this is the case, just take note of it and continue with your
    scan.

Open your awareness to the entire back and spine.

Many people experience discomfort in this area, as well.

If so, just acknowledge it and move on.

Bring your awareness to your face.

Take note of any sensations present here.

Move on to your nose, lips, eyes, cheeks, and jaw.

Sensations can be very noticeable on your face.

Maybe you feel a little itching, tingling, or prickling.

You may feel nothing at all. That's okay.

Now feel for anything happening with your ears, as well as the
    back and top of your head.

You may now open up your attention to the entire body and
    notice what it feels like.

Simply observe anything that arises.

You can return to normal waking consciousness. Both your mind
and your body will be feeling totally relaxed, and refreshed. If you
don't feel relaxed, that's okay. Keep doing it. It didn't work for me
immediately. I continued to practice until I started getting noticeable
results.

If you continue to practice this exercise, you will soon notice that
your awareness has increased. Staying in the moment allows you to
perceive those things that previously slipped under your radar. Your
relationship with your body will change as well. You will begin

paying attention to those subtle signals it sends to alert you to a potential problem before it becomes a full-blown crisis.

G. They Look Beyond the Solution

Problem-solvers look past the issues at hand to find opportunities. This means that uncovering the truth or hitting upon a solution is just the beginning. The meritorious problem-solver goes one step further. There may be hidden gems waiting for us after the answers become known. A person with a keen mind and an entrepreneurial spirit will jump on any lead that promises an extra thrill to the already successful outcome. There are infinite possibilities and probabilities that spring from every situation we concern ourselves with. Even though you have come to a solution, there may still be fruit worth picking. A worthy problem-solver can identify new avenues to take advantage of (in an honorable way). An example of this is a person terminated from a job she has been in for twenty years and has hated just as long. Her termination was a blessing in disguise. She now has the option of pursuing a career (or other interest) for which she has a real passion. This is like looking for the silver lining in a dark cloud. It's looking beyond a given situation. Don't bother trying this unless you are able to form a positive attitude.

The body's primary mandate is to be healthy. As a reminder, health care professionals refer to this desirable state as homeostasis. The body will seek out every opportunity to correct an imbalance. The body has its own ebb and flow of energy. This energy is always slightly out of balance. It oscillates like a pendulum to the right or left, moving back and forth in equal measure. When the pendulum swings too far in either direction, the body may become ill. This has

85

to do with the law of polarity and the law of rhythm. These forces are responsible for the rushing and retreating of the tides. Both laws govern the physical universe. The body seeks to maintain a natural balance within its systems and organs. Like all things, the body will always strive for a state of perfection, with the understanding that change is an essential ingredient to the recipe. Our bodies understand the natural order of the universe. They operate in harmony with those laws.

There are many alternative treatments available to help the body achieve balance. The methods I am familiar with require the manipulation of the vital life force. These **therapies involve the use of energy fields. There are of two types:**

Biofield or bioetheric field therapies manipulate the vital force that sustains our bodies. There are many names for this energy, such as universal life force, chi, orgone, prana, and vital fluid. Some of the more recognized energy therapies work by releasing and moving blocked energy. Though one cannot positively identify the source and nature of this mysterious force, energy healing is a popular alternative to western medicine. Examples of energy therapy include:

- Reiki
- Qi gong
- Therapeutic Touch
- Polarity Therapy
- Acupuncture

Bioelectromagnetic-based therapies make use of pulsed and alternating, or direct current electromagnetic fields, in an attempt to change the nature of the body's own electromagnetic field, thereby bringing about healing to the affected area. This approach is getting the attention of medical professionals for its successful application in the treatment of musculoskeletal issues. It has also proven useful in relieving pain. Those scientists involved in researching the medical uses of electromagnetic energy are beginning to appreciate the future it may have for the body's healing process.

A German physician named Franz Anton Mesmer, born in 1734, conceived a theory called "animal magnetism." Mesmer incorporated the idea of an invisible fluid and ordinary magnets to bring about healing in his patients. Even today, academicians and intellectuals regard Mesmer as a controversial figure (or a charlatan). Nonetheless, Mesmer's life and work greatly contributed to the development of modern hypnosis.

Transcranial Magnetic Stimulation (TMS) is a process by which inductive brain stimulation with alternating eddy currents neutralizes the polarity (depolarization) in the neurons of the brain. This exchange causes indefinable activity in certain parts of the brain. Researchers say TMS is a promising treatment for conditions such as Parkinson's disease, strokes, migraines, depression and some psychotic disorders. TMS devices were first available for treating patients with depression in October of 2008. A TMS depression study conducted by the Center for Advanced Imaging Research and the Brain Stimulation Laboratory at the Medical University of South Carolina has shown positive results. Their 2010 studies show that Repetitive Transcranial Magnetic Stimulation (RTMS) offers a certain amount of relief from the nagging symptoms of depression. It's conceivable that one day TMS will replace electroconvulsive therapy (ECT) also called "shock therapy" as the primary treatment for medication resistant depressive and psychotic disorders. I say this with the understanding that ECT is an entirely different treatment.[15, 16, 17]

TMS technology is still in its infancy, and it will be fascinating to see where future research leads.

H. They Achieve Lasting Solutions

True problem-solvers are not out to ease the symptoms of a difficult situation, they intend to totally erase the disturbance from memory. The problem-solver is idealistic. He seeks to return to a state in which the problem never existed. This is an excellent target to shoot for. Their attitude is full of merit. With determination, the problem-solver will achieve their goal.

Taking on a project with no intention of finishing it is illogical. This demoralizing behavior helps no one. It may even create a false sense of security, which invariably makes the problem worse. Rather than disappointing people, it would be respectful to stay away. If there is no lasting solution, the trouble will soon return. A permanent solution should be the goal of any problem solver. Leaving loose ends is not the mark of a professional or a person of integrity; such a policy leaves people unhappy. This leads to bad feelings all the way around.

Of course, it's a different story if you are unable to complete a project due to a serious illness or something beyond your control. No one expects you to perform miracles. Obviously, there will be times when we take on a project and soon realize that we are not the right person for the job. You may find that you are not happy with what you have gotten into and have become completely ineffective. In these instances, it may be time to get out of the game. The bottom line is that our sincere effort matters the most. Always do your best to create solid long-term results that consider the well-being of everyone involved.

The classic problem-solver is interested in an equitable solution. The problem-solver's goal is to arrive at an agreement that leaves all parties feeling satisfied. The idea is to make the outcome a win/win for all parties involved. It's always about doing the right thing and factoring in the needs of others when working through a particular matter. It's important to consider how your attitude and actions will affect the person with whom you are dealing. This sounds like common sense, but not all of us follow this rule. A purported solution that has hints of an "all for me and none for you" deal, or is otherwise imbalanced, is not a solution; it's more like a scam. A problem-solver knows that the course of his or her personal growth and development rests on the ability to deal fairly with others.

Our bodies expect that we establish permanent equitable solutions in our personal relationships. This lends itself to many of the higher personal qualities like integrity that help maintain homeostasis in the body. This philosophy keeps our bodies healthy. Operating outside of moral excellence leaves us feeling run down and discouraged. Our bodies urge us to be at our best. Leaving projects half-finished is not a good policy. How does this statement sound to you? "We have unfinished business to take care of." Not very pleasant, I'm sure. I think I've heard this line in a few gangster movies. Just knowing that we have something hanging over our head provokes a great deal of anxiety. The body reacts in much the same way. This a state of unease leads to many of the common diseases we face. Such uneasiness affects our mind body, and spirit. It's universal. There's just something satisfying about completion.

I. They Bring People Together

The problem-solver tries to bring everyone together. He knows that everyone must be on the same page and committed to creating a solution. Isn't it true that many modern day governing bodies, both corporate and governmental, require a unanimous vote for their decisions to become binding? An example of this is our jury system. Traditionally, you would have a twelve-person jury in a criminal trial. In 1970, the Supreme Court ruled that a six-person jury would be sufficient. In determining guilt or innocence, the jury must come to a unanimous decision. If the jurors cannot reach a unanimous decision, a mistrial may result. Coming together on an issue is crucial. No one should be unhappy with the outcome although more often than not someone is disappointed. That leads to a wide imbalance.

A good problem-solver garners the support of all involved. He will work hard to get everyone's participation. Here is another pertinent saying – "If you're not part of the solution, you're part of the problem." This means you needn't sit around and complain. Take action. Be a can-doer.

When human minds come together, they become part of the mass mind or mass consciousness, a collective entity, which is composed of the entire human population. The human mind is powerful and only increases its strength as other minds combine with it. Two can do so much more than one. The mass mind allows us to tap into the creative power and talent of virtually any, and all, sentient beings. You can do this by making an effort to gain their cooperation by bypassing their ego, and connecting with their minds on another level. On that other level, which I'll refer to as etheric, everyone is receptive and ready to assist you. Can you imagine having the complete and undivided attention of the entire human population? What do you think that would be like? That is the awesome power of the mass mind. A creative problem-solver or highly intuitive person can have access to the mass mind to bring about a resolution to a complex matter.

How does the body feel about this? The little minds are in complete agreement. There are no quarrels between our cells and internal structures. At times, it seems that the heart will argue with the brain or vice versa (our analytical unit and our emotional center). However, they are all working in unison. Most of the time, everything works perfectly. It has to. When there is gossiping and dissension between the little minds, we can expect things will break down. This can happen if super mind throws a monkey wrench into the harmony of our bodies. As you can imagine, this unwanted confusion gets the little minds frustrated to no end and leads to unwanted illnesses. Effective leadership will keep order in the body.

A worthy problem-solver sees the issues by taking on the other person's views. Truly, this step may be the only way we are able to resolve the challenge we are facing. When you are able to put yourself in the other person's shoes, you are at an amazing advantage. You are able to see through the other person's eyes. Not only that, but you are able to understand how that person thinks. You may be quite surprised at what their world looks like. It may be substantially different from your own take on things. Of course, when you understand the problem, you are now in an excellent position to conceive the solution.

How do we reach the point where we are able to get the other person's perspective? The answer is empathetic listening. This communication strategy involves comprehending the message the other person is sending, as well as the sender's intent and the circumstances surrounding it. Not only does empathetic listening allow the recipient to see the other person's views, but to live it out in his or her own mind. It's as if you connect mentally and/or spiritually with that person and gain an understanding of what that person is dealing with. Here are some benefits of empathetic listening:

- Empathetic listening builds trust in personal relationships through rapport.

- It gives you a greater degree of influence over a situation.

- It uncovers hidden information buried either intentionally or unintentionally.

- It will engender a sense of appreciation for what the other person is going through.

As you can see, empathetic listening is an indispensable tool for attacking a difficult situation. If you can't define a problem, how can you ever hope to have victory? Defining the problem always comes, in part, by seeing it from the view of the complainant. Even though we may think we know how something works, if our understanding doesn't relate to the other person's worldview it doesn't matter.

When I perform a criminal defense investigation, I interview everyone, including the defendant (my client). I want to hear it straight from the horse's mouth. They are your biggest source of information. However, their account may not necessarily be the most reliable. I found it's imperative to understand the client's mindset in order to be of help to them. This requires ferreting out the truth. The way to do this successfully is to develop a strong rapport, so that the information received is truthful and accurate.

Here are some tips for improving your empathetic listening skills:

- Be attentive at all times. Stay clear of any stray thoughts or distractions when he or she is talking. Practice this.

- It's important to keep yourself from forming judgments and opinions while the other person is talking. You may want to refrain from analyzing the speaker's message for the time being,

- Validate the speaker's importance by giving them your undivided attention. Maintain natural eye contact and display appropriate body language.

- Ask simple questions intermittently to maintain continuity and gain insight. You might also affirm the speaker's concerns now and then if appropriate. This lets the speaker know that you are interested in what he or she has to say. Use discretion when doing this.

- Try to be aware of the speaker's body language. This will provide you with the speaker's state of mind and the underlying meaning of his or her statements.

- Most all of you need to be quiet. Let the other person do most of the talking. You will get more information this way than if you interrupt with unnecessary questions every five seconds. My interviewing technique was to let the witness do all of the talking. People always end up saying more than they need to. This is in contrast to the famous line, "We'll do the talking" made by actors playing police officers in television dramas. Note that when you interrupt with excessive comments, the speaker loses his or/her train of thought. This results in poor communication and a lack of rapport.

You need to understand that this technique takes practice. The best thing to do is work on quieting your mind. This will keep you from speaking out of turn. Being human, we tend to think that everything we have to say is so important that we must get it out immediately. Relaxation exercises work well for this. Being patient will also help. I am no master of empathetic listening. I work at it just like everyone else who chooses this method.

How does empathetic listening relate to the body? As I have tried to emphasize throughout this book, whatever the super mind thinks directly affects the body. If you are able to train yourself to use empathetic listening in your human relationships, you can use it for better communication with your body. I told you there was a point to all of this.

Humans place great importance on having their concerns acknowledged, as do all creatures. The body likes to know you are interested in what it has to say also. Our bodies are always sending us messages. They all have specific meanings. Empathetic listening is the skill you need to interpret these messages. This is an essential skill in terms of your well-being. Ignoring your body's messages can have dire consequences. Try practicing your new listening skills in all of your personal encounters. Once you have become proficient with this technique, you will be ready to use it in communicating with your body.

Some basic approaches for using empathetic listening with your body are:

Pay attention to pain in all its forms. Pain is not normal at any time. I hear people dismiss their pain by giving uncertain explanations. "My back is bothering me. It must be old age." "I get headaches all of the time; it must be stress." "I get pain in my left leg. It must be that old football injury." All of these statements are excuses designed to avoid dealing with the problem. A lot of us do this. However, delay tactics do not solve anything. We only catch the body's signals to those matters requiring immediate attention, when we actively listen, especially to discomfort in all of its forms.

Do not criticize or blame yourself for perceived failures and mistakes. If you blame yourself, you are also blaming the little minds. This cuts off the internal dialog between you and your body. Your organs and systems will react to your mental assaults by withdrawing. Treat your body with the respect it deserves. Work out your emotional issues with a close friend or a professional, if necessary. It's essential to both your mental and physical health.

Show your body you are listening to it by taking action. Key messages from your body may include:

- Eating nutritious foods and following a realistic exercise routine.

- Losing vices like smoking, alcohol, and controlled substances.

- Engaging in inspiring and insightful activities like, meditation, prayer, yoga, music, dancing, art, gardening and hiking.

These nine qualities are the primary means for identifying a first-class problem-solver. This short list does not include other desirable qualities that may contribute to the problem-solver's character. Neither is it necessary to possess all of these traits to be regarded a problem-solver. You now have the tools to develop your own problem-solving mindset. It makes for an exceptional life experience. Your worldview will change for the better if you have the right attitude. Your problems will not automatically disappear just because you have adopted this mode, but your life will have an excellent outlook.

Autonomy

Self-actualized people are modest and respectful in their dealings with others. They prefer to be of service, rather than having others serve them. Even though self-actualizers may come from greatness or be famous in some way, their manner will come across as sincere and unassuming. A self-actualized person, no matter what their station in life, knows that all things are equal. Wayne Dyer in his book *The Power of Intention* points out that no person is special, even though our ego might tell us differently. The self-actualized person seeks to eliminate the special identity created by the ego, so that real spiritual development is free to take shape.

Being self-actualized is indicative of possessing an autonomous mind. It's just that self-actualized people desperately value their independence. In fact, it is sacred to them. They can conceive of no other way of operating. Self-actualizers do not thrive in societies that impose rules and regulations restricting self-expression. Their spirits must be free. Self-actualized people are often self-employed. That doesn't mean a self-actualizer can't work for someone else, either as a salaried employee or wage earner. The key is that self-actualizers like to be their own person and live life on their own terms. These entrepreneurs are accustomed to calling the shots. They hate being micro-managed.

Since America is "the home of the free," maybe autonomy is akin to national sovereignty. You could say (leaning on American civil liberties for support) that the signers of the Declaration of Independence were a mass mind of self-actualizers. The Declaration of Independence is rooted in our forefathers' intent to separate from Great Britain and have autonomy. In this case, autonomy became a statement of the natural birthright of each individual to be free.

In the Bill of Rights we find a number of specific autonomies. In the first amendment alone, we find the rights to religion, speech, press, assembly, and petition. These liberties are fundamental and form the prevailing belief system upon which this country rests. Even in business, the government has a laissez-faire policy of allowing private parties to be free from excessive regulation. It's debatable as to whether policy makers are sticking to the spirit of this principle. In any event, autonomy is clearly an essential liberty in the minds of world citizens. Self-actualized people do extraordinarily well in America. It's fertile ground for growing this distinctive breed. Nevertheless, other conditions must be present for an entrepreneur to succeed. There are many excellent sources of information on the various aspects of entrepreneurship. If you haven't guessed, this is an extra credit assignment.

In 1963, Erik Erickson conceived his Eight Stages of Development. In Stage Two, which occurs somewhere between eighteen months and three years of age, the idea of Autonomy vs. Shame emerges. At this stage, a toddler has a real opportunity to build autonomy. The toddler is learning many new mental and motor skills. They are also learning right from wrong. This is the stage where the child seeks to control his environment and the things in it. Here, you will see the mayhem of the "Terrible Twos." At this stage, the typical defiance, temper tantrums, and stubbornness appear. I trust that everyone has seen a child throwing a temper tantrum in a supermarket. Need I say more?

A well cared for child will use his newfound independence to build self-confidence. Autonomy is encouraged by offering the child choices. When you make a meal, offer the child two choices. Rather than telling the child that he has to eat broccoli for dinner, which he hates, offer carrots or some other alternative. Choices give the child a sense of self-control and builds confidence.

Children not given sufficient space to express their independence will learn to doubt themselves and their abilities. Stifling a child's autonomy at this age leads to shame. Children tend to be vulnerable at this stage, sometimes experiencing feelings of ineptness during a period of difficulty in learning new skills.

It seems that children may be a bit fragile after all. I can assure you that statement is true. If it were not true, I would not have been in business as a private detective for so many years. A large percentage of my cases involved clients and subjects having issues stemming from childhood that made them delicate emotionally and mentally. I'm not insinuating that such people are weak by saying this. Most things are beyond our control as children. Children depend on responsible adults for their well-being.

Now let's be adults for a moment. As I suggested earlier, you could compare our bodies to a top-notch corporation. When everything operates as it should, the company realizes a profit. A well-run company gives its employees its policies and procedures, and then the employees carry out management's orders. The employees know what to do and should have the autonomy to do it. Under the right conditions, this will work perfectly. My un-researched theory is that increased autonomy will allow employees to experience a greater role in the success of their company, thereby increasing job satisfaction and motivation. This results in better work performance and higher productivity.

Our bodies are thoroughly familiar with the idea of autonomy. There is autonomy within the organization of the body. The body is self-regulating. However, our bodies do their job independently of our conscious minds. Our bodies need no rigorous oversight from us to perform critical functions. In fact, it seems that when we get involved, without understanding the process, things tend to go haywire. Unless you are an architect yourself, would you tell one how to do his or her job? Some people would. We can all sleep soundly knowing the pros are taking care of our bodies.

Our bodies are well-designed machines with complex systems, and yet its members are autonomous. The body has a master network, which sends instructions to the body given to it by the brain, and therefore, the super . This powerful network is our autonomic nervous system. This system is divided into the central nervous system (CNS), which controls functions below our conscious awareness, and the peripheral nervous system (PNS). The CNS includes both the brain and spinal cord. The PNS includes sensory and motor neurons. The PNS includes the somatic nervous system (SNS), which receives all physical sensations, and the autonomic nervous system (ANS). The ANS is an involuntary system. It is concerned with the sensory and motor neurons that extend from the CNS to our organs. The ANS divides into the sympathetic nervous system and the parasympathetic nervous system, which regulate involuntary actions, such as heart rate, respiration, perspiration, salivation, digestion, urination, and arousal.

It may seem like a real paradox when I say that our bodies are working independently when, in fact, the body has its own control systems in place. For our purposes, these systems are autonomous, as our minds are not consciously involved in their day-to-day management. All organisms need a reasonable level of oversight or things get out of control. When people have 100% freedom, they do whatever they want. This isn't a good thing, which is why we have laws. Can you imagine what would happen if our internals did whatever they wanted? That's one reason for disease. We have systems to keep this in check. So my point here is that you can have autonomy in a well-regulated system. You have an assignment and management gives you the responsibility to carry it out. There is a considerable amount of autonomy present in this working relationship.

Activities go on in our bodies that are not visible to us. Our body's systems are flexible. Think about how our bodies deviate from their routines. In fact, our bodies may not even have established routines, as we know it. Our body's schedules change each day. They are far from being precise or rigid. Even our heartbeat varies. Yet it stays within the parameters set for it. That's the way our bodies are designed. Above all, this efficient organization works remarkably well.

Our bodies are of the opinion that there is nothing special taking place inside of you, although it is incredible to us. The little minds do not have egos. They are not looking to make their mark on the world. They have no need for incentives or benefits to get their jobs done. Our bodies do require solitude from time to time to get the rest it needs. The little minds need a vacation (in a manner of speaking), from the undue, mental, emotional, and physical stress that we put on our bodies. This happens when all of our organs and systems slow down, during sleep and rest. Again, it's fair to say that our little minds need what the super mind needs.

Spontaneity

Spontaneity is the state of being spontaneous. That's not a big surprise. This happens naturally and is not of external origin. Observing spontaneous behavior in people is fascinating.

Self-actualizers are famous for their charisma and charm. Their spontaneous energy is inspiring. Many people find the quick wit and lively conversation displayed by a self-actualizer appealing. People associate a spontaneous person with fun and excitement. These folks love the off-the-cuff humor and a sense of adventure that spontaneous people bring to personal relationships. Spontaneous people can be pleasantly impulsive. I had a friend once say, "Let's get on a plane and fly to New York City. The airfare is a bargain." It can certainly be an attractive quality. At the same time, it can also be bothersome to those of us who are not going at the same speed.

Self-actualized people have leadership qualities. They get people motivated, and are highly persuasive. Just for reference, I am not purposely trying to generalize here. I am just describing the classic self-actualizer. With self-actualized types, expect the unexpected. They will use their creativity whenever the opportunity presents itself. This, of course, goes back to their problem-centering characteristic. We often see spontaneous self-actualizers in the arts. Robin Williams is one of my favorites. I feel the comedians of Saturday Night Live are some of the most spontaneous entertainers I have ever seen, on or off the show. Many rock stars are incredibly carefree and spur-of-the-moment. Political leaders tend to restrict their natural spontaneity due to their position in society. They have an image to uphold. The public expects a politician's character and conduct to be refined and polished. It should be easy enough to find a self-actualizer based in part on their spontaneity. It could even be someone you know.

The body clearly enjoys moments of spontaneity. That quick energy increases the body's vitality. Our bodies are especially receptive to spontaneous energy. In fact, the little minds in our bodies are always stimulated, especially when the super minds are in sync with them. Our cells are already teeming with energy of their own. Spontaneity gives them that extra surge. It fires up the whole body. Chemicals are excreted that get the little minds, and the super mind, even more elated. Our blood sugar goes up releasing endorphins and other feel-good hormones into the body, getting everyone excited. It's as if someone gave us a million dollars (I wish). In any case, the little minds are experiencing a good time because of the surplus energy. Although it doesn't necessarily have to be a big rush, there could be a slight buzz feeling.

Appreciation

Appreciation is gratitude expressed toward something or admiration for an individual. This is not a dictionary definition. A self-actualized person always operates with a sense of wonder and awe. He has a high regard for life and every sensation. He expresses sincere gratitude for the opportunity to be here and fully experiences every moment. A true self-actualizer never takes life for granted, for he knows that someday he will not be here. Whether it's a walk in the rain, sitting in the sun, smelling fragrant flowers, or some other simple activity, the self-actualized soul never ceases to be amazed at what the universe has to offer. John Denver was a prime example of how to worship the wonder of life through the medium of music. My favorite is "Annie's Song." The use of similes in this song is beautiful. Denver exemplified the qualities of self-actualization. I want to remind you that attaining self-actualization does not make you a "perfect person." It's a special state of being that encompasses the qualities we are discussing.

The self-actualizer also knows that every experience is precious. This includes both the ones we label as good and bad. The truth is that we are here in this life to have experiences, learn from them, and bring this information back to the Infinite Mind. The Infinite is an ever-expanding energy or force (that's the best term I could come up with) that finds sustenance in the volume of experiences we bring back to it. Each new and unique experience contributes to its perpetual expansion. Our thoughts and emotions are especially valuable to the Source. Contrary to popular belief (in my view), the God does not know everything. At least it does not have knowledge of our personal interpretation of events in the material world. We are also permitted to enjoy ourselves in the process; otherwise, we wouldn't be eager to take part in this production. We are not that different from Pavlov's dogs in the sense that we are unusually susceptible to positive reinforcement to perform. It's for this reason that cosmic engineers created a sex drive in us, so that we would reproduce, and appetite so that we would eat. We do not like doing something unless it feels good. That's why we will leave a job where we feel unappreciated. People drift away from situations that they find unpleasant. Of course, people will still do things they don't like if they are pushed.

An appreciation of life is of the utmost importance. A self-actualized person looks for the beauty in others. She does not try to change them, for she knows that other people must change themselves and if they truly desire to do so. In support of this, our exemplary behavior should inspire others to be their best. If we do anything less than that, we are not operating with integrity. This positive attitude shows our gratitude for having these people in our lives. After all, we are learning from them. Be thankful for every person you meet, even if you are not particularly fond of him or her. Personalities of all kinds are assisting you in your personal growth and development. Praise be to God. I mean that respectfully.

We can all agree that our bodies crave recognition. This subject has been touched upon, but it bears mentioning again. If our bodies feel unloved, they will close up, and eventually break down. Our little minds are like any other living creature; they need acknowledgment, which comes out of love. We all need a certain amount of appreciation. This goes back to the need for love, which is why it's on the pyramid. If you are sick and want your insides to get back on track, I suggest you start saying encouraging words to them. It takes a thousand compliments to overcome one disparaging remark. That's a variation of one of Dr. Phil's famous lines. We seem to dwell on our seeming defeats rather than appreciating the good things already present in our lives. Society encourages us to express our displeasure and withhold praise. This practice destroys us from the inside out.

Words are thoughts manifested. Speech is more powerful than thought, and the written word is even more powerful than speech. When we aim our negative energy in the direction of another, it is likely to be picked up and absorbed into his or her body. Be aware of this fact when you become involved in a verbal exchange with someone. Sticks and stones may break bones, but names hurt even more. This statement is true for most people. It seems that someone got the original adage wrong. Words hurt, and they hurt physically. Speech can be a destructive force, especially to the body. The average person is not always capable of warding off such an attack. Go ahead and count how many times in a day you receive and transmit critical or unwelcome remarks. Observe how it makes you and the other person feel. It's a revelation. When you do this, you will see how much verbal pollution you are putting out and receiving. As a result, this exercise should increase your awareness of this issue. My hope is that you will become more guarded and protective of your mind and body, as well as what you send out to the world.

There are ways of talking to your body in order to give it all the encouragement it needs to flourish. Start with LOVE. Love is all you need. Love, love, love. You see all emotions are the offspring of love. This is a key concept. Even emotions like anger, hate, jealousy, and bitterness owe their existence, to love.

Think of the anger a dutiful parent might exhibit toward her young teen caught shoplifting. The parents will likely punish the minor in some way to prevent the dishonest behavior from reoccurring. The anger behind this action comes out of love for their child. It is very easy to recognize.

You'll find that even abusiveness is a twisted form of love. Still most people are only aware of the evil behind such heinous acts. That is understandable. Evil is nothing more than a distortion of love. To be sure, I'm not condoning abuse in any form. Let's consider another scenario.

When a partner cheats, the affair usually comes, as a surprise. After the unsuspecting partner gets confirmation of an affair; he or she will become justifiably enraged by the betrayal. You can see that this anger comes out of love. We are not making any judgments good or bad. We're just observing the truth as it is. Keep in mind, every circumstance is slightly different, so it's difficult to generalize.

If all emotions, spring from love, then what are we left to assume? Perhaps that love is all that truly exists in the universe. All things begin with love and end in love. Love is the alpha and the omega. You may choose to meditate on this and come to your own conclusions.

Many past and present day religions have attributed human qualities to "God." I do not mean to single out Christianity. The Bible is extremely inspiring and has some excellent lessons in it. It's just easy to for me to examine since it is part of my experience. The Old Testament portrays Yahweh as an angry and jealous God, given to violently punishing his beloved Israelites for disobeying his laws and defying his authority. Additionally, from the creationist story of Adam and Eve, comes the concept of original sin, in which all humans are born sinners. In other words, no one is worthy of God. Is this interpretation of the Divine accurate? I have my doubts.

Let's be clear that God, or Universal Intelligence, Infinite Source, cosmic mind, Collective Consciousness, is essentially a creative energy or force of pure love. One thing is certain; God made man in his image (God is gender neutral). We are a part of the Source through and through. We originate from and consist of this same love energy. God permeates the universe with this love energy. It encompasses all things that exist, both physical and mental. Yes, we are one, an immeasurable and indefinable energy. I can best describe this as pantheistic monism. I would ask that the philosophy scholars give me a break on this.

We have a unique love relationship with our bodies. If you love your body, your body will love back. As a result, it will cooperate with you. Therefore, you will be in a state of optimal health. Disease will be nonexistent. Love heals. You heard it here. Let me say it again for the people in the back row. Love heals.

Our insides have feelings. The various organs and systems have their own personalities. Love is just as vital to the little minds as it is to us. As with any entity in this vast universe, the little minds desire respect. This is a straightforward concept. Do you enjoy respect? Do your friends expect respect from you? The need for respect is a universal. It is highly prized by all living and nonliving things. To illustrate this intense pursuit, I refer you to the song "Respect", which became a phenomenal hit for Aretha Franklin in 1967.

What does respect mean? It means that your love for others compels you to use integrity in your personal affairs. You treat others, as you would like to be treated. Your body needs the same decent treatment from you. The little minds look for respect from the super . It's a case of mutual respect.

Imagine a disrespectful teenager. If you currently have, or have ever had, one of these temperamental youths, you should find this easy. Would you say their behavior is difficult at times? I'll bet that is putting it mildly. From the parent's perspective, teenagers seem to go out of their way to challenge us. Even if we don't have teens, we were all young at one time. Did you ever give your parents a hard time? We all did. Few of us can deny that we were, at the very least, a little mean and spiteful at some point. Is it normal? I don't know if it's normal, but it's certainly not acceptable. And, unfortunately, it's fairly common. Why do our teens do this, or why did we do it to our parents? It's lack of R-E-S-P-E-C-T. It could well be that the lack of respect is mutual. As I said, we all need respect. Let's be clear that self-respect isn't the same as respect. Respect is something we receive from other people. Self-respect is something we give to ourselves. We can't control whether people give us respect. To be sure, there are people who will criticize us, even if we are at the top of our game.

Many of us perceive young minds as being inferior and not worthy of our respect. Humans have a tendency to feel superior to all other life forms, as if they do not matter. We unknowingly do this with our teens and everything else in our environment for which we are responsible. Chances are if we treat our children this way, and our dog, our house, and our personal possessions, then we most likely treat our bodies with disrespect as well.

Our bodies react in much the same way as an angry teenager whose feelings have been hurt. This regrettable circumstance is the origin of many of our worst diseases. It's a vital point of which to take notice. As I said, our bodies answer all conscious and unintended messages received from our minds. It's a core component of the Body Alive Principle.

The mental applications discussed in this book are excellent ways for reaching the little minds. This is especially useful when you want healing. Visualizing is an effective method for accessing the mind, body, and spirit. Visualization is the application of intense mental focus, and directed imagery, designed to achieve a particular purpose. For our purposes, visualization is the primary vehicle for communicating with the little minds. Affirmative language aids in this process. Your mind speaks to the little minds using thought. They communicate telepathically.

What I am speaking of is the basis for every magical or psychic system, from ceremonial magic to shamanic journeying. Ceremonial and ritual magic uses visualization to complete evocations and incantation rituals to achieve their objective. Psychics employ visualization to attain altered states of consciousness, develop intuitive abilities, and contact spirits. Shamans use visualization to explore inner worlds. That's been my experience.

Visualization is gaining popularity as a tool for detecting and treating complex medical disorders. Visualization has successfully treated or cured almost every conceivable physical and mental illness, or injury. If an illness exists, creative visualization can treat it, and even cure it.

What follows is a short imagery exercise to relieve, perhaps permanently, the cause and effects of gastrointestinal diseases like Crohn's disease, inflammatory bowel disease, colitis, diverticulitis, and related disorders. I chose digestive disorders since my wife lives with Crohn's disease. The visualization script I am about to present is useful for any health issue. Just modify the template provided with the details of your condition.

Before I present this exercise, let's just review and reinforce a few ideas. Your body is its own best healer. Your body can correct any illness from a headache to a tumor. It may reduce the symptoms of the ailment or perhaps eliminate it altogether. What does your body do when it gets a cut? It will heal it. Our tiny cells are busy killing germs even as we speak. They do this without our knowledge. It's their job. It's what they've been programmed to do. They do this job better than any medical physician does.

Now let's consider the autonomic nervous system. This master control system is responsible for the following body functions:

- Circulatory
- Digestive
- Endocrine
- Immune
- Lymphatic
- Muscular
- Nervous
- Reproductive
- Respiratory
- Skeletal
- Urinary

The key to the Body Alive Principle is an understanding that our organs and their accompanying systems are aware of themselves and their role. The nice part is that we are never troubled by their everyday activities. We don't even have to think about it. All of the systems work behind the scenes to keep our bodies functioning.

In some cases, such as with autoimmune diseases, our cells get the wrong message and start attacking our organs. It is our responsibility to set them straight. Our bodies require our conscious supervision in these cases. Our bodies will listen to the super mind, in the sense that we have the final say at all times. There are documented accounts of yoga masters being able to lower their blood pressure, slow their heart rate, and raise or lower their body temperature.

So we agree (I hope) that every part of your body possesses its own awareness. You can look at individual body structures and individual cells as separate entities. It's fair to say that every atom in the universe maintains its own life and unique personality. Simply put, every atomic structure is alive. The Earth itself is a living organism. There is nothing new about this statement. Many ancient civilizations incorporated this idea into their beliefs and practices.

It's necessary for the successful application of this visualization that you accept the belief that your body is alive and can heal itself. We are trying to build a better relationship with our bodies. Our insides require even more attention than we give to our outside. The little minds respond to praise and positive feedback for doing their jobs. Think of what happens when an owner pays no attention to his or her puppy. I mean no patting or praise. Well, most likely the dog will get mean and lash out. The same thing happens to the human body. All of the individual structures in your body need nurturing. They deserve some credit. They are assuming an active role in your continued existence.

Please understand that I am not advising you to stop your current medical treatment in order to follow this method. It is perfectly acceptable to use this technique in conjunction with your physician's treatment plan.

If you have chosen to accept the ideas advanced by the Body Alive Principle, practice the routine that follows and you will certainly see an improvement in your health. Your body will respond to your commands and will begin the healing process. You should initially practice this method every day in order to achieve the desired results.

I like to start my meditations with a progressive relaxation exercise to put myself in a receptive state. You may choose some other technique to get yourself relaxed. There are many options. I do not recommend the use of drugs and alcohol as a relaxation technique. I encourage you to use this script or find a similar one on the Internet. You may also look for a book on stress reduction and practice the exercises or enroll in a relaxation class such as yoga or meditation. Use whatever method works best for you.

Progressive Relaxation:

Now we're going to get the tightness out of our bodies with this progressive muscle relaxation exercise designed to release the tension. It's fine to do this exercise either standing or sitting. Just do your best with it.

Start with your toes by curling them tightly. Hold for five seconds. Now release. Feel the tension escaping. Now relax for ten seconds.

Now flex your left foot and toes upward. Hold for five seconds. Release. And relax for ten seconds.

Flex your right foot and toes upward. Hold for five seconds. Release. And relax for ten seconds.

Tighten your thigh muscles. Hold for five seconds. Release. And relax for ten seconds

Tighten your abdomen. Hold for five seconds. Release. And relax for ten seconds.

Focus on your lungs. Breathe deeply. Hold for five seconds. Release. And relax for ten seconds

Make your left hand into a fist and squeeze. Hold for five seconds. Release. And relax for ten seconds.

Make your right hand into a fist and squeeze. Hold for five seconds. Release. And relax for ten seconds.

Flex the muscles of your left upper arm. Hold for five seconds. Release. And relax for ten seconds.

Flex the muscles of your right upper arm. Hold for five seconds. Release. And relax for ten seconds.

Gently arch your back if you are able to. Hold for five seconds. Release. And relax for ten seconds.

Shrug your shoulders upward. Hold for five seconds. Release. And relax for ten seconds.

Scrunch your face. Hold for five seconds. Release. And relax for ten seconds.

Purse your lips together tightly. Hold for five seconds. Release. And relax for ten seconds.

Hold your teeth together for five seconds. Release. And relax for ten seconds.

Stick out your tongue. Hold for five seconds. Release. And relax for ten seconds

Close your eyes tightly. Hold for five seconds. Release. And relax for ten seconds

Resume a natural position.

You will find that the tension has left your body. You should feel extremely relaxed. If not, close your eyes for a moment and focus on your breathing until you feel yourself loosen up. Now let's do the visualization.

Visualization:

You can do this visualization either sitting or lying down. Use whatever position is most comfortable. Do not rush through this exercise.

Slowly breathe through your nose three times to relax.
Feel your body melting into the ground. Take some time to
> visualize this. Feel yourself in a state of complete
> relaxation.

When you are completely relaxed, imagine your body standing
> in front of you.

Look at your beautiful body.
Accept this whether you believe it or not.
You are perfect in every way.
God has created your body to work perfectly.
All of the parts of your body work as a team with the common
> goal of keeping you healthy.

Every cell in your body does its job to keep you going.
Your body loves you.
Each part desires to make you happy.
Now look inside your body.
See all of your systems doing their jobs.
Isn't it amazing?
Realize that your body has its own awareness.
Every organ in your body has its own unique personality.
Every cell has intelligence right down to the very atoms.
Your body is a unified system with individual members working
> for your benefit.

Your body seeks harmony.
It wants to serve your needs.

Observe your internal structures busy doing their jobs.

Focus on the digestive system

This organic network is truly amazing

It is designed to keep you alive.

It was formed by the Divine Source to make your experience possible.

Now look at your intestines.

The large and the small intestines.

Look even more closely at the area that is causing you pain.

See it clearly.

What does it look like?

What color is it?

Praise your colon for doing its job so well.

Let your colon know that you appreciate it.

Tell your colon that you love it – say it out loud.

Send love to your colon.

Now ask your colon to repair the damage present.

Picture your colon healing itself.

See it healing before you.

You may feel your belly getting warm,

Or observe a sense of wellness emerging

See the tissues coming together and mending.

See the affected area disappearing entirely.

Now see the colon whole again as if it never had an injury.

What color does it have now?

Thank your colon for healing itself and making you feel better.

Tell your colon it has nothing to be afraid of from the anxiety you experience.

Tell it everything is fine and you are in control.

Again, send love to your colon.

When you are ready, you can now return to waking consciousness feeling refreshed and invigorated.

You are welcome to adapt this template to your individual needs. You can substitute any anatomical descriptive terms with the actual body part, organ, or function that is giving you trouble.

Template

Visualization:

Slowly breathe through your nose three times to relax.
Feel your body melting into the ground. Take some time to visualize this. Feel yourself in a state of total relaxation.
When you are completely relaxed, imagine your body standing in front of you.
Look at your beautiful body.
Accept this whether you believe it or not.
You are perfect in every way.
God has created your body to work perfectly.
All of the parts of your body work as a team with the common goal of keeping you healthy.
Every cell in your body does its job to keep you healthy.
Your body loves you.
Each part desires to make you happy.
Now look inside your body.
See all of your systems doing their jobs.
Isn't it amazing?
Realize that your body has its own awareness.

Every organ in your body has its own unique personality.

Every cell has intelligence right down to the very atoms.

Your body is a unified system with individual members working for your benefit.

Your body seeks harmony.

It wants to serve your needs.

Observe your internal structures busy doing their jobs.

Focus on the area of your body that is the source of your pain, discomfort, or symptoms you are experiencing.

The function this organ, system, or structure performs is of great importance to your health.

It's designed to keep you alive.

It was formed by the Divine Source to make your experience possible.

See it clearly.

What does it look like?

What color is it?

Go ahead and thank this area of your magnificent body for doing its job so well.

Let the organ, system, or other body structure know that you appreciate it.

Tell your body that you love it – say it out loud.

Now ask your body to repair the affected area.

See the area healing.

You may feel your belly getting warm,

Or observe a sense of wellness emerging

See your cells working to correct the imbalance that is causing your illness or injury.

See the affected area containing your illness or injury disappearing entirely.

Now see your body whole again as if it never had an injury.

What color does it have now?

Thank your resilient organ, system, or other body structure for healing itself and making you feel better.

Tell the restored area it has nothing to be afraid of from the anxiety you experience.

Tell it everything is fine and you are in control.

Send love to that area of your body.

Send love to your whole body.

When you are ready, you can now return to waking consciousness feeling refreshed and invigorated.

Please continue to practice this technique until you have achieved the desired results. You will find your health has improved, often within a short time. This method is also perfect for weight loss. That's just a little bonus.

Peak Experiences

Peak experiences are unmistakable. They create an awakening within us. Everyone has one of these at some point in their lives. Some people have many. It's a feeling of awe and joy. It transforms your spirit. This phenomenon is not exclusive to the self-actualized although they do have an attitude that is conducive to peak experiences. They have a rare state of mind that allows these glorious moments to enter their reality. People who are accustomed to these moments of wonder have open minds that are free from useless chatter. Self-actualized people have an intimate connection to the Universal Intelligence and draw their creative energy from it.

In my mind, a peak experience is more than just a moment of unusual clarity. This "feeling" comes to us as an awakening much

117

like a flash that goes off in our head saying, "This is magnificent!" In the event of a new idea, a person might exclaim, "By George I think I've got it!" Some people express their amazement by saying, "Yippee!" The peak experience is a natural euphoric state that allows us to see the universe in a special way. A woman I met years ago described her peak experience this way. She had been looking over a landscape and saw the sun sparkling on the leaf of a tree in such a way that it captured her attention. The spectacular sight mesmerized her. At that moment, she heard a heavenly voice say, "I love you." This extraordinary event changed her life. That is a peak experience. This is not the only way in which peak experiences manifest, and they do happen to all of us at some point.

These experiences seem to be random and unexpected. That is not the case, however. Self-actualizers look forward to these events as opportunities for both spiritual insight and inspiration. They do not *look* for them, however, as they will never happen when we want them to.

Peak experiences give you an altogether different perspective. They will alter your perception of reality. You begin to realize a greater force exists outside of the common reality. You may begin to question the reality you know. You may wish to seek the truth. You may already be on a higher path. This is a time for celebration and joy.

Uninformed individuals will try to induce peak experiences through artificial means, by using controlled substances like LSD and mescaline, as well as some designer research chemicals. While tripping with psychedelic drugs can be intense, it is not the same as a peak experience. By my way of thinking, a true peak experience does not occur in the brain. It is certainly a mind-altering experience though. Let's remember that there is a difference between the mind and the brain. The brain processes sensations from the body for the mind to experience. I am not of the opinion that drugs affect the mind; I believe that they work on the brain. Therefore, "mind-altering" drugs like mescaline (peyote) do not produce the same revelations you would get from an insightful meditation session. That's not to say that mescaline is a bogus method for achieving an altered state. It's just not the same as a genuine metaphysical event.

Mental illness can also produce a peak experience. With certain illnesses, the afflicted person will have epiphanies and moments of elation. These sometimes come across as extreme moments of religious fervor. This is due to brain chemicals like neurotransmitters not doing their job correctly. My feeling is that the mind is intact, but the brain is feeding it faulty information.

Peak experiences are frequently experienced by people with bipolar disorder. Medical professionals call it a "mania". This phenomenon is possibly due to an increase in the neurotransmitter dopamine, which may be responsible for the characteristic euphoria and behavior evident in mania. This is one possible explanation.

Based on this information, I tend to think that the mind is impervious to injury. Yes, it's true that the mind is easily influenced, and will oscillate in one direction or the other based on temporal experiences. It may even develop disorders such as Post Traumatic Stress Disorder (PTSD). However, the mind can never sustain permanent damage. It only appears damaged in this life. The process of mental illness also works in reverse. The originating PTSD experience can cause turmoil in the brain, creating episodes of extreme anxiety. We have much to learn about these disorders. I am certainly not a psychiatrist, and I admit that I cannot give a satisfactory explanation on such matters.

The body looks forward to these peak experiences. The minds of zillions of cells, and even the atoms comprising them, use such experiences to connect to the Infinite in a personal way. All sentient beings need to experience this divine union. They need to experience a part of that which is unknown. Humans especially need to know that they are a part of something much bigger than themselves. Peak experiences give us this hope. These memorable moments give us what we need to keep going. The little minds, especially, crave this state of splendor.

Self- transcendence

Self-transcendence is not included in Maslow's original pyramid. Maslow added a number of levels in later years, including cognitive, aesthetic, and transcendence. These additional levels represent our higher needs. While I want to stick with the original pyramid, I feel compelled to address self-transcendence because of its state of supreme illumination. There are many definitions given to the concept of transcendence. My favorite meaning has to do with losing the ego and becoming aware of one's self, as well as realizing the true nature of reality. At the transcendent stage, one will through a higher evolutionary process, experience a union with the Absolute Source. There is enough material written about transcendence to fill more than a few bookshelves. Self-transcendence puts us above the human condition. You could say that one surpasses the physical. We have reached a level where we are truly one with the universe. As a side note, Immanuel Kant is the historical figure credited with the development of transcendental philosophy in the west.

Some familiar transcendent souls include the Buddha, Zoroaster, Jesus, Moses and Akhenaton, . These avatars lifted up humanity, changing it forever. They became the living embodiment of the Universal Mind. The teachings they imparted to us had the same underlying intention. They sought to give us a quantum leap into a new way of conducting ourselves. Some of us are listening, while many are not.

When we are in the presence of a master, we know we are standing before the powers of the Infinite. It's a passive and peaceful force, which emanates from their inner being. Their dignity and sovereignty is unmistakable. They embody man's highest spiritual attainment and then transcend it. They go beyond the worldly.

Transcendence is an honor given to us at birth. At this stage, you have risen to the point in your evolution, where you are destined to become a great spiritual leader. You feel it inside you. It motivates you. For those of you chosen for this elevated position, hard work is the order of the day. Everything you do is in furtherance of the mission imparted to you by the Source. The transcendent master willingly and joyfully casts aside worldly ambitions to make way for this high calling. To be sure, the process for getting there can be arduous. We know this from the lives of Jesus, Moses, and other avatars. The physical world is not always kind to cosmic masters.

Transcendentalism

Transcendentalism is a movement thought to have come into existence between 1830 and 1860. Its leader was Ralph Waldo Emerson. Emerson sought to break away from the materialistic mindset beginning to take shape in America. Those versed in the ideals of transcendentalism view it as both a spiritual and philosophical movement. Taking its roots in Cambridge, Massachusetts, outsiders came to know this informal group of innovators as the Transcendental Club. Some of its members included Ralph Waldo Emerson, Henry David Thoreau, F. H. Hedge, Margaret Fuller, Theodore Parker, George Ripley, and Bronson Alcott. This

121

group looked to create a new spiritual and intellectual energy. The initiative they put forth certainly helped shape American literature. These influential figures came together due to their dissatisfaction with the societal values and religious doctrines in place at that time. Members of the Transcendental Club believed that the higher virtues of spiritualism transcended the lower physicalist mentality. They were certain that this higher state is accessible only through one's inner resources, including intuition. Aspects of these teachings have continued under other names and in other movements.[18, 19, 20]

Transcendental Meditation

The Maharishi Mahesh Yogi introduced Transcendental Meditation (TM) in the 1950s. The Transcendental Meditation program has achieved a global presence and is offering the Transcendental Meditation technique in dozens of countries. Its roots lie in the teachings of the Buddha, Krishna, Shankara, and Patanjali's yoga sutras. The benefit or aim of Transcendental Meditation is to experience the "source of thought" or "pure awareness." The pursuit of this ideal state prompted its leader to institute the International Meditation Society for the Science of Creative Intelligence in 1961. In 1971, Maharishi introduced the Science of Creative Intelligence, and a global expansion of the system was launched.

At the time of this writing, I do not have any experience with Transcendental Meditation, so I cannot rightly comment on the benefits and usefulness of this program as far as the Body Alive Principle is concerned. From what I understand about this program, its principles are characteristic of traditional meditation. Developing a better relationship with your body through meditation is essential to the philosophy of the Body Alive Principle. So in that sense, it may be helpful. The Transcendental Meditation Program claims the method will prevent and improve many common ailments including diabetes, ADHD, epilepsy, insomnia, anxiety, and depression. One of the drawbacks of this program is the cost, which according to some reports can run into the thousands, although you should check with Maharishi Foundation for the exact costs. If you cannot afford exorbitant fees for a meditation program, you need not worry. There are numerous meditation centers in every major city. Most offer their classes for next to nothing. Is it the same training you would receive taking Transcendental Meditation? I don't know. I encourage you to look into it.[21]

PART IV

Personal Qualities Necessary for a Healthy Body

"Honesty is the cornerstone of all success, without which confidence and ability to perform shall cease to exist."
Mary Kay Ash

Honesty

Honesty means being sincere and truthful. It also implies that one treats others fairly and is straightforward in his or her business affairs.

Why is honesty important to our bodies? Honesty is the mark of a noble character. The body has a strong need for us to conduct ourselves in an upright manner. When we treat others fairly, we enter into a loving relationship with them. The universal consciousness operates this way; so should we. Let me put it this way: do you believe God can ever be dishonest? No, the Infinite Consciousness always treats us fairly and with unconditional love. The secrets of the universe are available to all who care to seek them. Honesty is part of the universal order. It is something we can expect. Since the little minds thrive in this state, they have need of the super mind to operate this way. This allows us to be in accord with the natural rhythms of the universe.

Cheating is the act of dispensing with honesty in order to acquire something that would ordinarily not be available to us through legitimate means or would come with a price. Why is cheating a problem? Think of it this way. How well can corporate executives expect their employees to function in their jobs when their immediate supervisors act dishonorably by cheating and lying? It's obvious. Cheating never gets you ahead. It only gets you in trouble.

The principal reason why people cheat is greed. Greedy people do not recognize that their cup is bottomless. They do not comprehend the truth that the universe is abundant, and there is more than enough for everyone. Greed is a destructive force. It is a perversion of our basic motivations. Greed rears its ugly head when we are not satisfied with what we have. Societal deterioration is a reflection and manifestation of our overly materialistic attitude. I remember that the 1980s was a notoriously decadent decade. A friend of mine who was in a rock band summed it up by writing a song with the main lyrics "I want more. I want more." Madonna, the "material girl," covered the subject even better with a song by the same name. Not that it was such a terrible song. Greed consumes us. We look for happiness in material objects and activities. This leads to addictions of every kind and is extremely unhealthy.

I'd also like to add that there is no rational purpose in accumulating vast amounts of money just for peace of mind. We often develop our worst illnesses worrying about what to do with it. I'm certainly not against wealth. It's just important to have the right attitude. My two cents is this - it's reasonable and prudent to make financial plans and build a nest egg but don't think too far into the future, or should I say, don't *rely* solely on money for your future well-being. Circumstances can change overnight. Work on your resourcefulness, enthusiasm, motivation, and creative abilities to get you through the hard times. Don't forget about your hard-earned experience and natural talent. These personal attributes and resources will get you a lot further than cash in the bank. I live by this principle.

Look at this famous scripture. John 8:32 "Then you will know the truth and the truth will set you free." There are many ways to interpret this passage. I believe that for Christians, this scripture is concerned foremost with the truth in Jesus Christ being the savior of humanity. There are also metaphysical interpretations that deal with the pursuit of higher knowledge. I believe this message instructs us to seek a clean heart and spirit. For some of us, that may mean we need to "come clean". When we are honest we feel good, and it feels good to be truthful with others. Lying makes us feel dirty. Lying has several negative side effects:

- The lines between reality and unreality become, blurred, so that you are no longer certain of the truth.

- Lying tends to make a bad situation worse.

- You descend into fear and paranoia at the thought of being discovered a fraud.

- Guilt haunts the liar, and guilt can destroy.

- The longer the lie goes on, the bigger the consequences are likely to be.

Embracing honesty relieves us of these nasty effects. This reason alone should encourage us to be pure in our affairs. This comes from my own experience as a detective.

Lying includes bending the truth to get what you want. We need to go about doing things the right way to get our needs met. Cheating and lying are sure ways to fail at all your endeavors. Dishonesty can only sustain us for a short time. People will not tolerate dishonesty for long. People, who are dishonest, end up lonely and often destitute, wondering why they have not succeeded in life. I know there are many examples of people who cheated in life and seemed to do quite well for themselves. In the final analysis, did they really come out on top? Did they find success in more important areas of their lives? We don't know what goes on behind closed doors. In spite of their ill-gotten gains, their private lives would tell a different story. Some people have skeletons in their closet, and others have train wrecks. Don't ask me how you get a train into a closet.

Your body will react to such misfortune, ultimately affecting your health. It's like the domino effect in the sense that, when one aspect of your life goes wrong, the whole thing comes down, culminating in the compromise of your good health. When everything is going your way, you think you are getting away with it, but your body knows differently. This irresponsible lifestyle of cheating and lying will not go on indefinitely. Guilt always wins out. I feel I am qualified to talk about this. Most of my clients (and subjects) did things they wish they hadn't. They may or may not have been aware of what they were doing at the time. I'll be discussing true guilt in another section.

Many investigators are experts at reading body language. Investigators use nonverbal behavior such as body language to identify and ferret out the truth. When you lie, your body gives you away. The little things you do like twirling your hair, lowering your eyes, and folding your arms, are all telltale signs that you are not providing the whole story. These behaviors are relatively unconscious and almost involuntary.

Lie detectors (polygraphs) are another method for uncovering deception. They measure the body's responses and reaction to probing questions. Polygraphs will record physiological changes in heart rate, respiration, bodily movements, and the sweat glands. The polygraph detects sensitive body functions that reveal the subject's mental and emotional state, including the feelings that give you away. You see your body will not let you get away with anything.

Nevertheless, there are certain times when telling those "little white lies" or omitting the truth is acceptable. It may be appropriate to tell a fib when:

- When telling the truth would cause the involved parties unnecessary problems where none previously existed.

- The information needn't be volunteered, and the truth is of no consequence to the other person.

- Mental, emotional, or physical harm would come from its disclosure.

Example #1: An overweight friend is trying on a new dress, which doesn't fit her and she asks you how she looks in it. You wouldn't say, "You look amazing in that dress;" that would cause her embarrassment. Nor would you say, "It looks terrible on you," as that would lead to hurt feelings. Instead, you might say, "It's not your color," or "That dress is not the right style for you."

Is it a lie? Technically it is. However, it's the best solution to a difficult situation. Even if you said congenially, "You might want to find something that fits you better," you might start an unnecessary argument that creates bad feelings between both of you. Opinions have an uncanny way of taking on the appearance of the truth, and the truth can hurt.

Example #2: A friend asks you over for dinner. However, you already have plans with your cousin to go to the theatre. Your friend has a tenuous relationship with your cousin. Because of this, you tell your friend you already have plans. She presses you for details. And because you are backed into a corner, you tell your friend you have to work late.

You see this sort of thing in sitcoms. Is it a lie? Certainly it is. Can you get caught? Possibly you can. You have to decide which scenario is the lesser of two evils, being caught in a lie or hurting the other person's feelings. I believe other people's feelings are especially important. Some people believe in the absolute truth. Either philosophy is risky.

Do these examples go against what I am preaching? There are exceptions to laws, doctrines, policies, rules, and beliefs, even when such systems seem to give no way out. People typically see exceptions as either good or bad. These are my exceptions. You may agree or disagree. We are all entitled to our opinions.

As always, it's about doing the right thing. How do you know which choice is right? You just know. Your intuition will tell you if your mind is clear. Honesty comes out of this process. There are people who use honesty to hurt others. Then there are those who believe they are doing the right thing, but are simply not thinking clearly, or are deceiving themselves. Honesty is a noble quality. It's also crucial to our bodies, and our good health. I recommend you commit yourself to the practice of honesty. Give honor to your relationships by approaching them with an honest heart. Strive to be truthful in your affairs, but do not hurt yourself and others to achieve that end. In this world, the truth is not absolute. I have found the truth to be riddled with opinions and judgments. Therefore, I ask that you use reasonable care and discretion in showing the world your honesty.

There is one other point I'd like to make, and this may be yet another controversial statement as far as honesty goes: you do not want to do anything to hurt yourself. This means that if those in charge are burning witches at the stake, do not admit to being a witch, even if you are one. You do not need to sacrifice your physical, mental, and emotional health for your beliefs. Though the truth may set you free, it can also get you or those you love killed. People are not always going to be pleased to hear the truth. Don't expect someone to give you a bouquet of flowers when you bring them unwelcome news, especially concerning something you have done to them. That's why you are given the right to remain silent. I'm not just talking about criminal law either. I'm just saying that you shouldn't reveal anything that will be detrimental to yourself or someone else. I am not encouraging anyone to hide information. That would be wrong. You should report situations that are illegal or otherwise fraudulent. To be sure, I disagree with the argument that honesty is a black and white issue (as if you couldn't tell). Each situation is unique and multifaceted. There are infinite possibilities that arise out of even the smallest matters. You need to use both your reasoning skills and higher sense to get the answer in such instances.

Trust

Trust is a key feature of any successful relationship. Without trust, the future of a relationship is in doubt. Most relationships fail due to a lack of trust. A large percentage of marriages and romantic relationships end, due to infidelity. The trust issue is also broken over money matters when one person in the relationship is not being honest about household finances.

A teenager or young man may tell a woman that he loves her in order to get her to sleep with him. A substance abuser may borrow money from a friend under false pretenses in order to purchase drugs. It's no secret that these people do not intend to keep their promise. Their method usually does not include a preconceived plan. Most of the time it's just an ordinary lie designed to fulfill their short-term needs or desires. Often it's just an impulsive act, which can be likened to a crime of opportunity. It's something they do because it's convenient. Such a misdeed occurs when a teenager saying he will be home by 10 pm, does not return until midnight. The trust is broken here. The relationship between the teenager and his or her parents is strained. This is a real problem.

My experience with infidelity leads me to believe that a private investigator can do nothing to make a lousy situation any better. Hiring a PI has the potential to make a bad situation worse. If you have to hire an investigator because you suspect your partner is cheating, then your relationship has reached its end (although not always formally), because the trust is gone. Please understand what I am saying. It is difficult to repair a relationship in this condition. Even if no betrayal has taken place, the relationship is still in trouble because the belief of infidelity is there. This unremitting thought of infidelity, eventually, becomes the gospel truth in the mind of the anxious mate, whether or not it is actually happening. If the targeted cheater discovers an investigator has been watching him or her, that fact becomes another nail in the coffin for the relationship.

Trust is an integral element of any relationship. We could not maintain our society without trust in one another. In fact, our relationship with the Infinite Spirit is based on trust. We have to know that the Infinite would never do anything to hurt us. The Universal

Spirit wants what is best for us because we are a part of its essence. Although terrible things seem to happen to us, we still trust in the Absolute Source. We often get angry at the Source for our circumstances, but we always seek out divine intervention in desperate times. If we cannot trust our creator, then we are without hope. The creator cannot forsake its children. The Source rarely destroys one of its members. It loves all creation. Every atom is precious. Therefore, trust comes from love and cannot exist apart from it. God is love.

Our bodies depend on us for many things, including leadership. Is it necessary to trust our leaders? Yes, but sometimes we can't. Understand the little minds feel this way about the super mind. We are confident in our leaders' abilities, so long as they do the right thing. When something goes wrong, and the super mind fails to handle a particularly difficult situation, the body breaks down. The trust between the little minds and the super mind is essentially broken. Our bodies expect us to manage the major events that we face each day. We have the decision-making role. Whatever we do affects the rest of the intelligent units making up our exterior. They *depend* on us, to manage our affairs with integrity. If your body becomes distressed due to your poor choices, bad habits, or outright neglect, it will let you know. Rest assured you will not like the outcome you receive.

Genuineness

When you are genuine with others, you are showing them your authentic self. This means putting on your real face for the world to see. The world does not want to see another phony. I take a dim view of fakes. I can spot them before they even open their mouths. They have a certain look that gives them away. Genuineness is a virtue I appreciate. My advice is to be yourself. My brother is extremely genuine, almost to the extent that it hurts him. He likes to keep a biker image complete with tattoos and leather. This is how he sees himself and how he chooses to present himself to the world. Everyone who knows my brother feels very comfortable around him. My three sisters also have attractive personalities that make them special. They are not afraid to be themselves, and they accomplish this by being friendly and sociable, which is how genuine people come across (for the most part). A genuine person shows his or her human side. It's not usual for people to bury this high-quality feature beneath feelings of animosity, bitterness, and resentment. Genuineness is more than just unleashing your feelings. It means exposing yourself to the world. This can be a tough row to hoe for anyone.

I'd like to note that genuineness doesn't mean you should be rude and obnoxious. I'm not proposing that you go out and treat people with disrespect. I can hear some of you saying, "Yeah, but that's who I am." That's not true. If your name is Moody Judy or Polly Put-off, you're the exception. In all other cases, we should endeavor to use our finer attributes. In my mind, genuineness is an act of respect for other people. People want to know our true selves. No one needs a facade or masquerade. There is too much confusion in the world already. As gentle individuals, we should endeavor to keep ourselves from adding to the problems of the world.

There are times when this kind of genuineness can work against you, such as at work, churches, schools, and other places having codes of conduct. There are times when society expects you to play the game, as with employment interviews. You have to put on a suit and act the part. If you don't do this, your peers will pass judgment. Appearances, count for more than personality, especially in the affluent nations. There are plenty of arguments in favor of the dress code and careful grooming. One of these is respect for the individual or organization you are dealing with. Some would call this etiquette "conformity". Living in a civilized society places certain expectations on us. In this modern age, there are times when conformity is necessary. This is what we have to work with.

Your body subsists partly on your genuineness. Much of this goes back to homeostasis. Insincerity throws your body's finely tuned systems off (although the human body is amazingly resilient). This is because you get out balance by being untruthful. In your subconscious, you know when you are operating from a bad place. In effect, you create a mental condition, which changes your body chemistry. Your body responds by allowing depression and anxiety (among other things) to take hold. There comes a point when the little minds can no longer withstand the baser mental transmissions of the super mind. As I said before, if you are interested in the metaphysical nature of matter and energy, you may want to pick up a book on the law of attraction. My wife tells me that the Abraham-Hicks books are very good.

Kindness

The Universal Mind is a loving and kind entity. It always treats us with kindness, even at those times when in human terms, we may have been less than deserving of it. The way we treat people is a reflection of our creator. Kindness is powerful—not a weakness. It takes a virtuous man or woman to be kind to someone who doesn't return that kindness. True spirituality requires us to show kindness to others even if we think the other person doesn't deserve it. This is in opposition to the Old Testament God who can arbitrarily withhold love as a form of punishment. The Universal Spirit is all love. Love is its nature. Therefore, it cannot withhold kindness from its offspring. We should extend this same expression of love to our fellow man. In a remark often made by Christians to those in a moral dilemma, "What would Jesus do in this situation?" Clearly, there are biblical teachings I agree with and Christian dogmas that I find offensive.

There is a difference between putting your needs first and being selfish. It is okay to ask the Cosmic Source to meet our needs and have those things that we truly enjoy. However, the creator does not want us to hurt others in the process of getting what we want. Selfishness and greed degrade our society; kindness elevates it. Kindness creates a better feeling among people and improves our lives. When we extend our kindness to others, especially those in need, it helps to spread the kindness expressed by the universe. The Universal Intelligence has given us abundance, so we have more than enough of his (I do not believe our creator has a gender, but I use the word out of convention) goodness to share with others. The Infinite wants us to share our kindness with one another freely and joyfully. The Infinite will not force us to be kind or compel us to give of ourselves. Kindness comes as an act of freewill. It has to come from our hearts, just as love from the Source comes freely to us. The Infinite Intelligence always shows us its kindness, especially when we are in need. So be kind to others especially when they are most in need.

Kindness is an act of love. It is not self-serving. We do not need to get anything out of it. True kindness is pure because it comes from the Source. By growing in kindness, we grow in spirit. As a result, our personality develops its finer qualities. As we practice divinely inspired kindness, we will experience and receive the same from the Infinite, which will change us internally. This change will express itself outwardly (externally) toward others and will be a healing force for those receiving this higher vibration. Healing is a physical

136

manifestation of kindness. Kindness creates physical changes in our bodies. It is conducive to physical, mental, and spiritual healing; i.e. healing the whole person.

Our bodies respond quite favorably to kindness. This is because the Cosmic Source embodies this quality, as I previously mentioned. The body seeks to align itself with the higher vibrations in the universe, by putting itself in harmony with its rhythms. Once again, this process falls into the domain of the law of vibration and the law of rhythm (Be sure to do your homework. Universal laws are important to understand, especially if you are into self-help). Our bodies are unable to attain this higher state when we withhold this same kindheartedness to our fellow man. Once again, I encourage you to do as your spiritual master would do. When we operate with compassion and gentleness, our bodies feel the ensuing soothing energy travel throughout their systems. This natural outflow of energy from our acts of goodness leaves the body in a state of pure tranquility. It turns out that kindness is beneficial to everyone at every level of existence, from top to bottom.

Empathy

This involves identifying with another person and understanding where that person is coming from, especially their feelings, views, motives, attitudes, etc. We have already discussed em*pathetic* listening, which is, in simple terms, is the purposeful and deliberate practice of listening to the other person with compassion and understanding. Empathy entails connecting with one another on a deeper level.

Developing a rapport with the other person is paramount, not only to get along with him or her, but also to bring unity to the relationship (whether romantic or non-romantic). When we do this, we not only gain an understanding of the person's circumstances, but we come to appreciate the person's true self. This goes beyond appearance and reputation. When we come to know the person's inner being, a divine union forms; one, which we may not be aware, exists. By learning to use empathy on this plane, we become kindred spirits, thus coming to know one another in a deep and meaningful way. Empathy is a powerful tool that can transform any relationship. A state of excellence emerges in any relationship when an empathetic personality is a part of it.

Once more, you do this by seeing the world through the eyes of the person you are communicating with. It's a melding of souls. This is especially important in romantic relationships. You can be so close to your mate that it may seem you know what he or she is thinking at times. It's possible to know the deeper aspects of your mate that would otherwise not be revealed. Empathy allows you to see things that go way beyond his or her beliefs and values. Identifying with your mate strengthens the bond of the relationship. It's this special insight that makes the relationship click.

As I discussed in the section on empathetic listening, our bodies work extremely well with empathy. Empathetic listening is a sure way to reach the countless sentient beings that inhabit your body. Rather than waiting for them to come to you, offer a listening ear. This is itself a bold invitation. Try to relate to your body and understand it. Relate to your body on its terms. Think on a cellular level. Use meditation to quiet your mind. I also recommend using creative visualization as part of your routine. By doing so, you will allow the Divine Source to work through you, and, therefore, the little minds.

Gentleness

Gentleness is a strong, compassionate quality. Many powerful kings and leaders have possessed a gentle nature. In the U.S. and many other industrialized nations, a gentle disposition equates to weakness. The uninformed consider a person of gentle nature to be inferior. These same individuals consider a highly competent person to be someone who possesses an aggressive nature. Aggression is even encouraged in some cultures. These societies believe that if you are gentle, you cannot be an effective leader. Of course, this is faulty thinking.

Remember, our greatest leaders were, above all else, men and women of gentleness. Just look at the lives of our transcendent leaders – the Buddha, Jesus, Mother Teresa, Gandhi, and Martin Luther King Jr. Some people will debate the status each of these leaders should receive. However, each of these masters shared a common characteristic. They all possessed a gentle spirit, which considerably enhanced their leadership ability. They were also beings of peace. Peace is "a state of mutual harmony between people and groups." Peace is the quality of gentleness, and vice versa. Our Source dwells in a perfectly peaceful state and desires the same for us.

A gentle spirit naturally supports a healthy relationship. A healthy relationship is one that creates "an emotional connection between people that promotes well-being." Healthy relationships are ideal for creating a condition of peace, love, and happiness. They feed us and keep us alive. They are also crucial to our survival. We need each other in a way that supports our physical, mental, emotional, and spiritual needs. Negative relationships sap our energy and can destroy us by creating disease. We need positive relationships that give us strength. Can you peacefully coexist with a partner who is constantly criticizing and berating you for everything you do? This may qualify as abuse. Is there any gentleness involved here? I don't think so. Can you see how a gentle personality would eliminate this nonsense and foster a relationship based on personal growth? We need to be good to each other to get to where we want to be in life.

The body requires gentleness to maintain its intricate operations. It will take only so much abuse before it quits on us. You may have heard the expression "Be gentle on yourself," or "Be good to yourself". Therapists use words like these with their clients. This phrase means what it says. Go easy on yourself. Beating yourself up over external events doesn't do your body any good. Negative self-talk can even make the situation worse.

Self-Control

One definition for self-control I like is, "strictly managing one's desires, emotions, impulses, and actions through the use of one's own willpower." Self-control is not to be confused with control, which is a power struggle with the Infinite. That being said, let's look at control for a moment. When one thinks of control, thoughts of government agents and police officers may come to mind. Many people associate control with power, which is partially true. Power is a delicate matter. When you assume a position of power, you also accept the responsibility that goes with it. In the Bible, God gave Adam power and control over the Earth, but he apparently had trouble doing his job.

Society's most influential figures often misuse their power. Tyrants, dictators, and oppressors use fear to control other people. Tyrants use fear to get others to do what they want. They play on your fears. Bullies possess no real power. They only retain and exercise the power we willingly give them. Playing on fears is instinctive to them, even when they don't know your fears they are still able to get to you.

Less-considered abuses of power include deprivation and fear of punishment. Any veiled or passive use of fear can be traumatizing. It can lead to feelings of lack and worthlessness. This treatment often leads to long-term emotional problems. In spite of this, we need to understand there are degrees of control. Some semblance of order is necessary in every society. Without some measure of control, we would descend into anarchy. People need regulation. They look for it.

Control and Illness

Sometimes people will develop serious illnesses to get attention, especially from their parents. Yes, I know I sound mean. I can hear it now, "Why would anyone do this to themselves." No one would *knowingly* take on a serious illness to get attention." However, awareness has many levels. I am not a psychologist, but I've seen it in more than a few people, and people operate in many of them at different times. I'm sure this happens in the subconscious where we are not aware of its existence. That is the nature of our psychological traumas. Many people who believe they are unloved somehow develop serious diseases. Medical professionals are not always able to track illnesses to their source, while others are relatively easy to trace.

Anorexia nervosa is a good example of the tie between food and emotional needs. Anorexia is an eating disorder that often starts out as normal dieting to improve physical appearance. However, even when a target weight is reached, the dieter continues this weight loss practice until he or she almost stops eating altogether.[22, 23, 24]

There are many contributing factors to this dangerous condition. A starvation diet may have its roots in control issues. The anorexic may feel that the only thing he or she has control over is his or her body. This is a sense of powerlessness in the world. Anorexics try to compensate for this lack of control by restricting the intake of food to their bodies. You see it feels good to say "no." The anorexic also gets measurable results from the scale. This is approval.

This extreme dieting behavior (if you can call it that) ultimately leaves the anorexic frustrated, angry, and depressed. The pain and isolation that comes with anorexia can be overwhelming, but weight-loss will never improve a negative self-image. The physical damage caused by this unsafe behavior far outweighs any short-term benefits. Anorexia leads to death in many cases.

Bulimia nervosa is similar in nature to anorexia. The most distinguishing characteristic of Bulimia is binge eating followed by purging; typically accompanied by other improper methods of weight control. Bulimia, much like anorexia, has its roots in control issues. This disorder comes with a distorted body image as well. A combination of anti-depressants and therapy is the usual course of treatment for this illness. I realize that the one-size fits all approach does not apply in psychiatry.

A relatively rare and lesser-known mental illness is Munchausen syndrome. Rudolph Erich Raspe made the name famous in the book *The Surprising Adventures of Baron Munchausen*. Karl Friedrich Hieronymus, or Baron Munchausen, was a German-born Russian military man living from 1720 to 1797. The Baron was renowned for telling tall tales about his supposed adventures. Baron Munchausen's reputation for his fabricated exploits gave rise to the name of this disorder.

This illness induces the afflicted person to invent diseases and injuries in order to secure the attention and sympathy of others. They "want" to be seen as a sick person. On another level, Munchausen sufferers believe their sanity can be regained through the respect of others and control of their outside circumstances. Since their lives have become unmanageable, this is not possible. The same things we all desire.

What's scary about this disorder is that these individuals will risk their lives by undergoing potentially dangerous operations and tests to achieve their ends. Some of the unnecessary tests and treatments are not only risky, but cost insurance providers tens of thousands of dollars.

Researchers believe that Munchausen syndrome has both biological and psychological aspects to it. After a thorough examination and the absence of any physical explanation for the patient's complaint, frontline physicians will often recommend the patient consult a psychiatrist. Once again, the treatment of choice for Munchausen syndrome is a combination of medication and therapy. As with most psychiatric illnesses, this disorder is extremely challenging. Any proper treatment plan will require a devoted professional to see it through. Any noticeable improvement in the patient's condition will take time to manifest.[25]

Then there are those who self-mutilate by inflicting injury or pain on themselves. This includes cutting the skin with a knife or razor until there is bleeding. Burning the skin, typically with a cigarette, is also common with self-mutilators. Medical professionals refer to this heartbreaking behavior as deliberate self-harm. This heartbreaking behavior is typical of borderline personality disorder (BPD) and some other mental illnesses. BPD has its own symptoms and features that sets it apart from the other disorders mentioned here. I encourage you to read up on it. The DSM-IV-TR Diagnostic and Statistical Manual of Mental Disorders is the clinician's reference book. This may be a good place to look if you are interested in how a professional determines this condition.

Self-mutilation is common in females (especially older children and adolescents) who have had a history of physical, emotional, and/or sexual abuse. Self-mutilation appears in people who grew up in families that limited emotional expression. Reports indicate that self-mutilation does not usually last into adulthood. It's estimated that up to 100,000 people at any given time in America intentionally cause injury to themselves. Self-mutilators typically suffer from intense feelings of powerlessness. Usually, the injuries are superficial, and there is no intention of suicide. In this case, the self-mutilator is not seeking attention. In fact, they tend to hide their wounds from others. As with anorexia and bulimia, self-mutilation is a coping mechanism. Self-mutilation is a method for releasing emotional pain, and for penetrating emotional numbness. Self-mutilators release the pain of their childhood traumas through cutting and burning. If a particular instance of self-mutilation does not fall under the category of a major mental illness, talk therapy can be an effective treatment option.[26]

Can the Body Alive Principle help with psychological conditions such as these? Absolutely it can. Getting in touch with the little minds will bring an understanding of what you are doing to your body. It also addresses the "whys." The Body Alive Principle brings the reasons for self-inflicted pain into focus. Facing the truth is a significant step towards healing. Examining your thoughts and feelings gets to the heart of the truth. Letting go of any attitude that takes your body for granted or treats it like an old suit, puts you on the path to self-realization. There is no outside competition to be concerned with. This is an internal battle, and one that's worth fighting. In that same breath, I'll say that it's not a battle *per se*, but it does appear that way, as you will discover. Getting in touch with yourself helps, you master your life. Peace lies at the end of the tunnel for those with the patience and persistence to do the work.

This discussion on control goes back to my earlier comment on reacting and responding to everyday occurrences. I'll repeat myself for extra measure. Self-control has to do with how you change yourself to cope with the different situations you encounter, especially those involving other people. Moreover, the Cosmic Source of all understanding does not wish for us to manipulate others in an unscrupulous way. When we try to control others or change them in any way, we are exercising a form of misguided manipulation. We all need to relate to, and behave toward, one another in a positive manner. It may seem impossible, but by seeking guidance from the Infinite, we are able to get the clarity that we seek.

Remember, stress is a reaction to a situation. It is an internal controversy; caused by our futile attempts at controlling someone, or something that is beyond our influence. It is not our job to change another person. Focus on what you can do to change how you feel about the difficult situations you encounter. I promise that if you do this one little thing, you will change your life, and dramatically improve your health.

Integrity

Integrity is adherence to a strict moral or ethical code. In my mind, integrity is of the highest value and summation of all other positive personal qualities. It's much like reaching for perfection in that we must continually strive to attain this impeccable state.

Our reputation is another person's opinion of our character. Our character is a reflection of our integrity. Therefore, your integrity defines you. It reveals the best in us. People will either respect us or disregard us based on the distinct character vibes we send out to the world. People known to have a good reputation will have an easier time in life and enjoy it more fully. Keep in mind, not everyone views integrity as a positive attribute. There are people who despise the "goody two shoes" for the way they carry themselves. The truth is, maintaining an excellent character in spite of ridicule, is our ticket to a better life. And we can feel good about ourselves too. I realize that exercising integrity in our professional and personal affairs is not always easy, given the corrupt state of the mass mind. It takes a person worthy of these qualities to do it. Thankfully we're all worthy.

Integrity is a state of being complete. When you have integrity, you are right with the Source. You will feel peaceful. If you violate your own integrity, you will find yourself unbalanced and moving away from the source. You may also feel guilty. With some exceptions, sane people do not like to feel guilty. People rationalize their behavior to justify their actions. All sorts of negative behaviors are justified by those living dishonorable lives. In the end, however, all negative behavior runs counter to real integrity.

You can't have integrity if you are not true to yourself. When you deviate from the path of truth that you have set for yourself, you will find yourself in trouble. Standing up for what you know is right is vital (you don't have to die for your cause, however). It's a rare person that can say he or she is entirely immune to the temptations and influences of the world. It is up to each of us to learn how to handle these situations. This is the reason core beliefs play such a central role in our lives.

There are no shortcuts to circumvent the integrity issue. It doesn't pay to take the easy way out. I'd like to point out that there are no get rich quick schemes. The only ones getting rich are the ones selling their shameless product or service to the unsuspecting public. I witnessed this repeatedly over the course of my previous career. This greedy behavior is what gets us into our predicaments. Just remember that when you create problems for yourself, you also cause problems for others. Our behavior always affects those around us.

It usually requires a significant shift in our thinking to bring awareness to our destructive behavior. Bad habits and negative behavior patterns are never easy to break. Deep down, we all know whether we are behaving the right or the wrong way. For most of us, integrity means listening to our inner voice. Some call this our conscience. Your conscience tells you when you are hurting or victimizing others.

Your core beliefs need to be in order so that you may act honorably. If your beliefs are not right with the world, your thinking will be faulty. Core beliefs are your operating system much like Microsoft Windows is to the PC. When a virus infects a computer, it will not function correctly. The same is true of our belief system. If something "infects" our thinking, it will profoundly affect our core beliefs and therefore, our behavior. The people who raised us instill their beliefs in us at young age. The people who played a role in our growing years also contributed to our belief system. If your personality is unappealing and unattractive, just look at the people and events that shaped it. We absorb all these negative experiences while young and do not understand that these events are the cause of many of our adult problems. For some people, dysfunction is a way of life, at least until a friend, teacher, or counselor guides them in changing their beliefs. Re-examining our beliefs is the first step towards an amazing recovery. This includes beliefs we hold about disease.

Our bodies respond strongly to our emotional expression. The body, like everything else in the universe, is emotionally driven. The body reflects the intensity of our emotions, in an equal measure.

You'll find that the little minds take notice of our moral and ethical violations. It creates a terrible feeling in us, perhaps in our subconscious. It's also possible to feel it physically. Some people feel it in their guts. Where it's stored, is unimportant. The important thing to take notice of is that, every time we violate our integrity, we lose another piece of ourselves. This happens when we fail to consider the impact our actions have on ourselves and others. This negative behavior creates a hardship for everyone that falls victim to our careless lies and deceptions. What may be even worse is the harm we cause to those people connected to the victims. The pain inflicted on the victims also causes us to re-experience the guilt of our irresponsible behavior. Additionally, our lies hurt us just for making them, and then the trouble the lies cause, hurts us again. It's like paying exorbitant interest on a credit card for something we bought two years ago. There's another life saving tip for you.

As I stated, integrity is the highest ideal. When our sense of integrity is solid, we are closer to the Source. Our bodies need this connection too. They operate best at this level. Therefore, integrity is central to the survival of the body. Our connection to the Universal Mind depends on adherence to high moral values. *That does not mean you will be shut-off, just because you had an impure thought.* Most of us are guilty of harboring less than honorable intentions towards our fellow man or woman at one time or another. That's the human condition. The divine allows us to learn from our supposed mistakes and improve on them. We talked about how we are evolving. In life, we pursue integrity. Integrity is not a state of being faultless or beyond reproach. Much to the contrary, we must constantly work at being the best we can be. The pursuit of integrity is much like the quest for the Holy Grail, but in a real way. It is not a fable, but it *can* be elusive. I will say it again - we are human. Therefore, we must continually correct ourselves and resume doing what is right. Just for reassurance, I, myself, am working toward everything discussed in this book. No creature is an exception to the universal laws that govern this material.

Illusion of the Body

PART V

Guilt and the Body

"A life spent making mistakes is not only more honorable,
but more useful than a life spent doing nothing."
George Bernard Shaw

Our bodies will need forgiveness to maintain homeostasis. Our bodies have a seamless connection with our minds. Our mental state dictates the health of our bodies. They are inseparable. An ill of the mind is an ill for the body. If the super mind accumulates harmful feelings such as guilt, the little minds will adjust themselves accordingly to reflect this state. If you your thoughts are spilling over with regret, the little minds will react to this negative distress with depression. If you find yourself overly stressed, they will react with anxiety. These are simple examples of course. Stronger emotions may elicit reactions even more severe than the ones I just mentioned.

There are levels to our mental states. It seems that the deeper the level, the greater degree of illness. Deep feelings of resentment, hatred, or bitterness may lead to a breakdown of the organs. For example, it's commonly accepted that heart health is negatively affected by extreme bouts of anger and hostility. Emotionally charged memories release cortisol into our bodies. Cortisol is a steroid hormone produced by the adrenal gland. Its main purpose is to increase blood sugar. Prolonged exposure to stress causes the release of cortisol, which can cause extensive damage to the body, including compromising the immune system.

Forgiveness is an integral part of the healing process. Forgiveness is the primary tool for bringing ourselves out of a downward spiral. If we can forgive ourselves for our past indiscretions and our perceived failures, we can count on restoring ourselves mentally, emotionally, and physically.

Before I go any further, I should point out that there are different types of forgiveness relative to our own healing. There is forgiveness by others, forgiveness of ourselves, and forgiveness by God or the Universe, depending on what term you prefer.

Forgiveness by others is not always necessary for our healing, seeing as victims (not just victims of crimes) do not offer it in abundance. This is unfortunate since expressing forgiveness speeds up their own healing.

Forgiveness by the Divine Source is easy, since the Divine is not capable of harboring resentment. This is because our life force had its beginning in the Source, and loves us unconditionally. The source cannot reject its offspring. Such a rejection would be akin to hating itself and this is not possible since all of creation would simply cease to exist. It almost sounds absurd.

Forgiveness of ourselves can be difficult due to the intensity of the guilt we are harboring. Guilt holds us captive. This can be a condition of society, as well as our religious upbringing. Most people in America are familiar with the Christian tenet that if you sin and do not receive God's forgiveness, you go straight to hell. I'm simplifying the matter quite a bit for the purposes of this book, but that is the essence of it. My theory on this (yes, another theory) is that Christians do go to a place like the biblical hell, because they have a guilty conscious over things they have done in this world. They also go there because they believe in it. People who amass feelings of guilt and deep regret for their wrongdoings in their lifetime may feel deserving of eternal damnation. It truly is a terrible fate and unnecessary. The truth is we tend to be our own worst critic. Just realize that the cosmic consciousness itself does not have to forgive you for your misdeeds because it holds nothing against you in the first place. There is only love both within and without.

By its own nature, guilt has long roots that burrow deep into our subconscious. Because the roots of guilt go deep, it is especially difficult emotion to remove. Guilt is an unpleasant and unreasonable customer. It has a rather pigheaded personality. In most instances, a person is unaware of the depth of their guilty mind. As a result, the guilt-ridden person will go through his days feeling fatigued and thoroughly distressed. Our bodies create this unfortunate condition as a reaction to the guilt. The little minds may feel they are under attack. Their work, now disrupted, leaves them unable to perform at an optimum level. The super mind is sending the little minds a signal they cannot work with. The little mind works best when attuned to the transmissions of super mind. I am not just speaking of the conscious mind, but also the greater mind. Guilt interferes with this finely tuned process. Guilt is an unusually strong emotion. It can overwhelm and even immobilize us. To free of useless guilt, we need to gain forgiveness. Specifically, we need to forgive ourselves.

There are all kinds of offenses, wrongdoings, misdeeds, crimes, sins, and indiscretions. Did I get them all? I am not judging them or labeling these acts. All matters have equal standing for the following application. Here, you will find a simple, yet powerful process for dealing with difficult, emotional issues that will bring balance to your mind and body:

Awareness (of the situation) – In this case, awareness is understood to mean, acknowledging what you have done to others. Put another way, awareness means looking at how your actions have affected others. As a result of this new awareness, you might say to yourself, "Oh, I didn't realize I did that." It's as if a light goes on in our head. This might happen after years of being in the dark about an event, or even a whole series of events. For some people, this first step never happens. It may just be ignorance (I don't mean that in a derogatory way). Frequently, people push these incidents to the back of their minds because they are too painful to deal with. Subconsciously, the guilty pretend such things never happened. Bringing these events into the light will bring up guilt, and it may be something we prefer to remain hidden from us. However, it's necessary to face this emotion and subdue it in order to move forward.

Sometimes our guilt has nothing to do with a wrong we perpetrated against another person. This is what I refer to as a "false guilt." This flavor of guilt serves no useful purpose. False guilt regrettably leaves its victim's dwelling on terrible (or not so terrible) events we believe we had a hand in and had some control over. "True guilt", reminds us of our deviant behavior, and (hopefully) helps us improve our conduct. This guilt is only useful until it has served its purpose. I have chosen not address the topic of false guilt at this time due to my intentions for this book. Numerous self-help books on the market have sufficiently tackled this subject.

You may have encountered this concept at some point in your search for answers. Other authors have presented this information using different terms and explanations. I am not claiming to offer a novel idea. I am just presenting a new way of using it.

Acceptance – This means you are taking the situation "as is". This is when you look at your offense (you should examine them one at a time) and say to yourself, "This is what happened and I can't undo it." We can't go back in time and make changes. As the saying goes, "It is what it is." Don't try to make macaroni and cheese into a steak dinner. I know some of you like macaroni and cheese, but you get the idea. Acceptance is the idea that you realize the damage has been done, and there's no going back. You're not ignoring the situation; in fact, you're seeing the light of day. Simple acceptance often resolves our guilt. I'm not saying it is always that simple though.

Ownership – This is taking responsibility for the situation. You say to yourself clearly and with certainty, "I did it." It doesn't mean playing the blame game, "It could have been Bernie," or, "It could have been the weather." This is unconditional ownership. You're saying, "I take total responsibility for everything I did." If you had cohorts involved, let them take responsibility for whatever they did. Realize that their mess has nothing to do with your personal dung pile. Your body needs to feel your sincerity. It's a sweet relief. It takes some of the pressure off your body, and because of this, you won't feel so weighed down by your guilt. Therefore, by admitting our guilt we begin to feel better. That's why in some churches, you will see people stand up in front of the congregation and confess their sins. It's tremendously powerful. Don't worry, I'm not asking anyone to make a public confession. That's not necessary. Just be honest with yourself.

Atoning (for your transgressions) – This involves righting the wrongs *as best you can*. Do your best to restore the other party to their former condition. Sometimes it can be as easy as saying "I'm sorry." Other times it may take considerable time and effort. Just remember that you are not Jesus and cannot revive the dead. When we do our best to make things right, we may experience a sense of wholeness, as we are showing our honesty and integrity to the injured party. This should not be a painful process, although it could be a difficult one. It's a step towards freeing yourself from guilt's bondage.

Renewal - This act takes place when you make the decision to turn over a new leaf. It's a new beginning. This comes after completing all the steps previously mentioned. When we reach this stage, we choose to turn our backs on our former life. If you think you have never done anything wrong, you may disregard that suggestion. However, speaking from my own experience, there is always room for improvement.

Renewal is a spiritual awakening, not necessarily in the Christian sense, although it could be. Our light shines at this stage. We have learned a valuable life lesson and a new way of thinking. Renewal gives us the opportunity to show the world our best. If you have had a renewal of the spirit, you have chosen to align yourself with the Infinite. You have made a divine connection with the Infinite Source from which you came forth. You have developed awareness that you are part of something bigger than yourself. A feeling of joy may come over you. This feeling will carry you out of any obsessions about guilt and inadequacy. It's a sense of freedom, and it is life changing.

This is a safe, reliable method for freeing yourself of stubborn and worn-out guilt. This approach could be the exact thing you need to lift yourself out of the mud. It's a straightforward process, although it's hard work. You can get help and encouragement from your family and friends, if they are willing to give it. Bear in mind this is a journey of the spirit; you must make it alone. These journeys are always extraordinary.

We all start at the bottom and work our way to the top. When we're at the bottom looking up, it may seem intimidating and even fearsome. We've all been there at some point. The Bible points out that we are all sinners (although I see that in a slightly different way). We have all done something we are not proud of. Most of us have had, at least one significant event, which has given us acute psychological stress. It doesn't even have to be a major incident to give us a heavy dose of guilt and regret, since we all interpret our experiences in our own way. Many of us have never gotten over those events.

After completing your hard lessons, the little minds need you to release any unnecessary and unproductive feelings of guilt. They cannot continue to exist in an environment of harshness and self-reproach. Can anyone live like that? Is it necessary for you to dwell on your disappointments, defeats, failures, mistakes, and wrongdoings, as you imagine them, for all eternity? It's a miserable existence. Remember, your body is fulfilling a critical function. Your body feels what you feel. Do you want your body to feel badly about itself? Self-loathing is a terrible, terrible internal state. You need to release these harmful emotions right away.

You now have the option of climbing out of your pit. Do your best with this. There is no one competing against you. There will be no accolades or trophies for finding your back. The only thing you will get is the chance to hold your head high again. Is that worth the extra effort we must put into it? Say yes!

Illusion of the Body

PART VI

Trauma

"Happiness is not something ready made. It comes from
your own actions."
Dalai Lama XIV

The American dream has created a success-driven culture that encourages overachievers. As a result, we put high expectations on ourselves. Much of this is because we accept the expectations others place on us, even if they are unrealistic. We have a fear of disappointing others and a longing to be included. We also want to avoid looking bad. Therefore, the "average Joe", is determined to live up to the expectations others have set for him.

For the most part, we are all people-pleasers, busy trying to make our friends and family happy. There are people who will do anything to get a kind word and a pat on the back. This creates yet another undesirable condition.

Too often, people work through their lunches and put in extra hours in an effort to win the favor of their bosses. They regrettably neglect other parts of their lives, compromising their health and close relationships. No person can maintain a chaotic life for long without breaking down. The body isn't built for such abuse.

When people fail to live up to the expectations of others, a state of inner turmoil ensues. Feelings of failure rise to the surface of our awareness. The negative thought, *"I'm not good enough"* begins to establish itself as a belief in us. We accept this belief as an accurate representation of what is true about ourselves. Consequently, we birth emotions to go with this negative attitude like our wayward children: fear, regret, and guilt. These exact emotions give rise to depression and anxiety. That doesn't come as a big a surprise. Nothing pleasant or constructive ever comes from unrealistic expectations.

If you are one of these people, you may not even be aware that this internal state exists. Our mental commentary is usually just a blur. You can't even catch one word of it until you slow down. This negative input takes possession of our psyche and proceeds to establish itself as our basic programming. Our subconscious mind accepts it, not knowing the truth.

If things are not going right for us, we can assume we are working with negative programming that we have unintentionally allowed into our subconscious. This unproductive chatter, may be giving us suggestions like "You are a failure," "You should be ashamed of yourself," "You deserve to be punished." The list goes on and on. It's like an unrelenting rainstorm. It's easy to feel helpless against this overwhelming force. We've all been there. We've all experienced this to some degree.

A traumatic event is a little harder to deal with than getting a parking ticket. That's not to say that a parking ticket can't be traumatic for some people. I'm just addressing the "common man" for simplicity's sake. Psychological stress can occur in other forms besides a one-time event. Maybe someone mistreated you as a child. I hope not, but it happens. Perhaps you are a victim of the US mortgage crisis that reared its ugly head around 2008. There are no judgments coming from my end. Or maybe you had to put your baby up for adoption, I don't know. There are many such situations that we can become involved in that cause us mental and emotional distress. This can be the sudden loss of a loved one, becoming a crime victim, getting involved a serious accident, or anything else imaginable. These examples are all terrible things for anyone to go through. Even having a phobia of turtles (especially ninja turtles) can be a disabling to some people. All worries and concerns are valid.

At one point or another, we are all bound to experience a traumatic event. It's bound to happen. Inevitably, we will all experience mental or emotional pain. Pain comes in different forms, the most obvious being the psychological and physical types. Here, I am concerned with the psychological. Sometimes these events are so vivid and intense that they produce what is known as post traumatic stress disorder (PTSD). PTSD is an anxiety disorder. It involves re-experiencing the emotional pressure of a disturbing event, often through flashbacks or nightmares. This condition is prevalent among military veterans who have seen the horrors of war, although anyone can fall ill with this disorder.

Traumatic events are highly persistent and overwhelming. They are like large, frightening, mosquitoes that keep coming back for one more bite. No matter how hard you try, you cannot shake the awful recurring images that accompany the feelings behind them. It's unsettling, to say the least. The acute anxiety a person experiences from a traumatic event or multiple events can become debilitating. This means that a traumatized person is unable to deal with their day-to-day routines or function normally.

Another application of the Body Alive Principle is the technique used to relieve us of the painful recurring images we experience related to traumatic events. The Body Alive Principle uses the same principle for all diseases. It always regards the recipient, your body, as a separate entity and attempts to open a dialogue. An important piece to this involves *listening* to the complaining party (the little minds). The little minds desire to be heard. You must give them the attention they require to keep your body running properly.

Many years ago, I was experiencing my own psychological crisis, with the chatter in my head cheering on my feelings of failure. This episode went on for some time until I became depressed. This situation didn't stem from a single event, but from an ongoing series of deals, gone sour in my professional life. I took these events to be failures at the time. As a young man, I tended to be impulsive and reckless. I didn't think before doing. I recall my wife saying I have an entrepreneur's mind. My experience has shown me that there are a large number of entrepreneurs in need of direction. I have found that entrepreneurs have a propensity for getting caught up in the moment. It gives them a bit of euphoria. I'm not saying that all entrepreneurs are like this. Fortunately, I was able to temper my need for stimulation with a bit of self-control.

Without boring you with the details, I was worried about my career, finances, health, relationships, and everything else connected to me. It was a global sense of disappointment. The real failure was in not putting these events in the proper prospective. I had the idea that, for something to be successful, it had to conform to my high standards. I should have realized that not everything has to come out my way to be of value. My expectations are not the measure of success from the Cosmic Intelligence's perspective. I was stubborn at the time. I decided that this whole period was so utterly important that I had to dwell on each of my apparent failures until I got sick.

It is difficult for anyone to be around a depressed person. A despondent mood affects others in the household. Pessimism is catchy. If you have a problem at work, you will soon have a problem at home. Soon enough the bad feelings will begin to build, except now they will affect your close relationships. This makes for an unhealthy environment.

Our house, which itself is an entity, began to share in our despair and reflected it in equal measure. Our house produced all sorts of new problems for us, which are beyond the scope of this book. Our financial situation was one of the more obvious symptoms from the "bad vibes" permeating the house. We were living a relatively good life on money we didn't have to spend. We knew we had to change the energy in the house, which seemed to have turned against us. If you find it difficult to accept the idea of a house having its own personality, look into it, you will be surprised at what you learn. You will find each house has its own "air." A house seems to take on the personality of its owner or former owner. Some houses may seem sad, while others are quite pleasant. There are even houses that become openly hostile. This is the case with some haunted houses. I am speaking of the houses themselves, not the disembodied spirits that possibly dwell within them.

My wife thought we needed to deal directly with my mood as if it were a person. Had this been a single acute episode, we would have given the event its own name. My wife came up with the idea of naming my persistent mood "Charlie." We discovered that certain thoughts, and emotions, especially the baser energies, will at times, assume a physical form. People have described the manifestation of these emotions, as the proverbial dark cloud. These shadowy energies will occasionally appear to ordinary people. With our understanding of the situation, and knowledge of emotions existing as sentient beings, we theorized we could communicate with this negative energy using the Body Alive Principle.

I proceeded to have a conversation with this mood. I asked it why it had come. I didn't ask why it had come to torment me, but just "why." The answer I was given had to do with the story I recited earlier about my perceived failures. This made sense. Through careful listening and concentration, I learned that thoughts of my painful experiences had invited the mood. Nonetheless, I continued my dialogue with it. I asked exploratory questions. The mood responded accordingly. I asked the mood whether the reasoning upon which it based its presence was a true and accurate representation of what had taken place at those times. The mood and I went through each experience examining the reality of the event. This exchange required attentive listening to comprehend the mood's arguments. At no time did I insult the mood or blame it for my health problems. I sympathized with the mood's position and rationale for its presence. In the end, I asked the mood if it would like to go inhabit another place, as this space would no longer suit its needs. In a short time, the dark mood lifted, and I was able to go on with my life. In truth, I used very little persuasive language in this dialog. I spoke in a positive tone. I did not suggest, insinuate, or imply to the troublesome entity that it should remain with me, nor did I encourage its attitude.

Things that were disturbed in my life seemed to go back into place after this trying episode. That is the way of the Divine Spirit. When we change our attitude, we see our reality change with it.

By treating the mood as an equal, I was able to understand it and eventually, in a respectful way, encourage it to seek a new home. I didn't try to drive it out, since these entities will only dig their heels in. They have no real interest in moving out, unless there is nothing for them to feed on. Yelling at them does not do the least bit of good. These types of entities are much like parasites. They subsist on our negative thoughts. If you continue in this state, they will stay put.

When you have discussions with these beings, they may not respond with a human voice. Perhaps you may hear them as your own thoughts replying to your probing questions. That's fine. As long as you successfully resolve the matter, who cares how it is accomplished? In this book, we're looking at the outcome and working backwards. That way we know what we're getting right from the start.

Epilogue

"I have fought the good fight,
I have finished the race,
I have kept the faith."
Paul the Apostle
2 Timothy 4:7

To sum up, if you are good to your body, your body will be good to you. This may sound trite, but it's true. The body is an incredibly advanced machine, yet it's more than that, because we each occupy one. Our bodies allow us to experience our own personal reality. For that reason, I can safely say we have a close relationship with our bodies. If you wish to have the time of your life in this physical world, then you must do it in a healthy body. That means treating your body with gratitude and respect.

The entities that make up your body are very much alive and in need of your guidance. Leadership is a skill we must possess to be successful in all of our endeavors. A "take charge" attitude will carry us out from under the weather to soar above the clouds. Our employees, the little minds, follow the direction of the super mind. Whatever we experience is what *they* will experience. Be an exemplary role model. Show the little minds how to conduct themselves. This does not mean we will necessarily be able to do this on a level of reality that we can objectively perceive. Choosing to keep a positive outlook increases the likelihood of things going our way, especially in terms of health; and in other areas of our lives. As we know, the little minds respond extremely well to an upbeat attitude.

Above all, you must strive to keep your integrity. I should point out that failure is not an option if you should you fall short. You must pick yourself up; dust yourself off; and get back in the saddle. Determination shows the world what you are made of. We are spiritual beings having a human experience. By doing our best to keep up our integrity, we become human beings having a spiritual experience.

It's vital that you listen to your body. This means taking notice of the obvious signals like fatigue, soreness, nausea, and various types of pain. This is your body warning you that something has gone awry. Houston, we have a problem. You can become sensitive to your body's subtle messages by practicing empathetic listening. Try listening without judgment. See the topic of discussion from the other person's point of view. Use affirming language when responding to the other party. This practice will carry over into your communication with the little minds.

The little minds communicate in a psychic manner (for lack of a better word). Consciousness, or pure awareness, uses the mental nature of non-physical reality as a platform for a kind of communication known as mental telepathy. Telepathy is the usual form of communication between nonphysical beings. It may be the only method. In the physical world, humans use speech as the principle form of communicating. Therefore, we are able to communicate with less than 1% of life forms that exist in the universe. In fact, we are not even aware of the multitude of animate and inanimate things around us that possess consciousness, and intelligence for that matter.

One way to counter this shortcoming is to develop our intuition. Intuition allows us to perceive those things that are not apparent through our five senses, including many messages from our body. We may become aware of things that would otherwise remain hidden from us. We often experience a "knowing" just in the nick of time. It's remarkable. It may come to your mind as pictures, words, symbols, etc. Sometimes the universal consciousness steps in and you may even receive the answers in physical reality as visions, dreams, signs, ideas, inspirations, and miracles.

The best method I know to develop our sixth sense is through a consistent meditation practice. Meditation puts you in touch with your inner self. Getting quiet allows all those critical messages to come through to your objective consciousness. Mindfulness meditation using the body scan method is an excellent place to start. It may be difficult to maintain a regular practice in the beginning, because of a hectic lifestyle, restlessness, intrusive thoughts, and other mental impediments. They are of no concern. Keep at it. Success comes with gentle determination. "Actually, I'm an overnight success. But it took twenty years." – Monty Hall. I am just kidding. It just takes a little patience. You will eventually establish a routine that works with your individual challenges, rather than trying to thwart them.

Bringing your creative imagination into your healing meditations will give you the results you are seeking much faster. Visualizing the impaired parts of your body and seeing them heal is an effective strategy. Do this with your affirming self-talk. Communicate with your cells and organs in this manner to get the answers you seek. You will want to do this in a warm and caring way. Treat your inner beings as allies. Ask them to identify any problems that exist. Ask them to make their needs known to you. Your intuition will help you receive their reply.

In addition to all of this, I have provided you with the following fundamental principles necessary to keep your body working at its optimum:

- An introduction to problem centering and the qualities of a successful problem-solver.

- The personal attributes necessary to maintain a sense of balance between your mind and body, especially a strong sense of integrity.

- A process for healing your "true guilt," which will assist you in your pursuit of self-actualization.

- A technique available to you for overcoming psychological trauma.

You now have the knowledge and abilities needed to live a better quality of life. A new world has opened up to you. You have at your disposal all the tools needed to overcome illness and begin a loving relationship with your body. This effect will travel into your greater environment, improving your personal relationships, and ultimately enabling you to live a happy, healthy life. You can't prevent bad things from happening, but you can change your perception of these events, thereby conquering them. Developing the skills outlined in this book will help. Don't give up. I want to emphasize that we are all meant to achieve great things in life. Enjoy the journey.

All the best,

David

Appendix

Warning: Not for Human Consumption

While this section doesn't directly relate to the application of the Body Alive Principle, I feel it is necessary to bring attention to the fact that there are substances being added to our food that may not be safe. I will explain how these chemicals poison our bodies. Please read on.

One thing you can do to keep your body happy is, to be choosy about what you put into it, and what you keep out of it. Would you knowingly feed your body poison? There are many chemicals put into our food products that are not healthy and do nothing for our well-being. I'm not going to belabor the issue of proper nutrition. However, I am going to touch on some of the major chemical culprits that are slowly killing our bodies today. Since I am no expert in biochemistry, I have gathered relevant information from outside sources, which I think are helpful.

I realize these sinister chemicals are in most consumer foods. That makes them difficult to avoid. I am not asking anyone to stop eating their favorite foods in an effort to act on this information. Many people cannot afford to pursue an organic lifestyle. Others have health issues that require them to follow a particular diet. That's okay. This section is meant to bring awareness to the situation so that we can make informed choices. Use this knowledge to that end.

Sodium nitrite

Sodium nitrite is a preservative that is present in many of the processed meats we eat, like hot dogs, bacon, ham, and lunch meat. It is unusual to find sodium nitrite in fresh meats. Sodium nitrite gives meat the red color people have come to expect. For example, beef should be red, since it is a red meat. Warm-blooded animals have a protein in their muscles called myoglobin. Myoglobin appears as a dark grayish-purple color. However, when myoglobin combines with oxygen it's converted into oxymyglobin. Oxymyoglobin has a deep red color. Vacuum-packed meats are not exposed to oxygen and therefore do not turn red. Meat that is sold in special clear packages does not allow air to get through; thus giving it that familiar red color. Again, sodium nitrite preserves that color. Do not base the quality of meat on its color.

The American Institute for Cancer Research and the World Cancer Research Fund in their report "Food, Nutrition, Physical Activity, and the Prevention of Cancer: a Global Perspective," indicate a strong link between the consumption of nitrite-treated red meat and colorectal cancer. Cured meat is thought to create a carcinogenic effect after being cooked.[27, 28, 29, 30]

Sodium nitrite is linked to the following health conditions:

- Consumers may be at an increased risk for several types of cancer, including colorectal.

- Sodium nitrite has the potential to trigger episodes in migraine sufferers.

- One study indicates that the onset of chronic obstructive pulmonary disease (COPD) is linked to sodium nitrite.

- There is a possible relationship between sodium nitrite and brain tumors in children. Incidentally, the federal **Food and Drug Administration** requires retail packages of sodium nitrite to bear the warning, "Keep out of the reach of children."

High Fructose Corn Syrup

High Fructose Corn Syrup (HFCS) is a sugar substitute, not to be confused with artificial sweeteners such as aspartame (NutraSweet and Equal). Other names for HFCS include *isoglucose* and *maize syrup*. HFCS is corn syrup, chemically altered to turn its glucose into fructose. HFCS is found in hundreds of consumer food products too numerous to list here, but include breads, cereals, and soda. I recommend reading the food labels. Interestingly, as I write this, a news segment announced that the Corn Refiners Association is petitioning the **Food and Drug Administration** to allow them to change the sugar substitute's name to "corn sugar." They feel the name high fructose corn syrup gives it a bum rap. They want consumers to know the product is perfectly safe and natural. It seems to me a hamburger is still a hamburger by any other name. It's crucial that we be informed about what we are eating. The name high fructose corn syrup is a little misleading in that it is a kind of sugar, and many people do not recognize that fact. For that reason, changing its name to corn sugar makes some sense. Then consumers would be able to identify it as a sugar product. On the other hand, I would be somewhat concerned that this would be giving consumers a false sense of safety. Calling this genetically modified food product corn sugar does not make it safe. Being that HFCS is so prevalent in our foods, there is reason to be concerned. Allow me to elaborate on this point.[31]

As previously stated, much of this research relies on information found at the websites listed in the footnotes:

Obesity

There have been numerous studies, which show that HFCS consumption leads to obesity. When you put excessive amounts of sugar into virtually every consumer product made, you are asking for trouble. Some organizations push HFCS as a "natural" substance. You might have heard recreational drug users pitch marijuana as a natural substance. I realize HFCS is not marijuana; I'm just pointing out the absurd arguments people and groups will make to justify their position. Organizations like the CRA assure the unwary public of the safety of HFCS. This misinformation encourages consumers to ingest large quantities of HFCS-containing products. I am convinced that our fondness for HFCS is lethal. I do not make that statement lightly. Many people have an addiction to HFCS that, in many ways, is similar to other chemical dependencies like alcoholism. We know obesity leads directly to serious health conditions like:[32]

Cancers - endometrial, breast, and colon	Liver disease
Dyslipidemia - elevated cholesterol and triglycerides	Respiratory issues
Gallbladder disease	Sleep apnea
Gynecological abnormalities	Stroke
Heart disease	Type 2 Diabetes

Hypertension

Fructose affects blood vessels by reducing the availability of nitric oxide. This is significant because nitric oxide relaxes the blood vessels and thus lowers blood pressure. Since fructose hinders the production of nitric oxide, blood vessels cannot relax and dilate normally.

Another way HFCS can cause high blood pressure is by increasing the amount of uric acid in the blood. That is a signal to the kidneys to eliminate a dangerously low level of sodium. This situation leads to other problems in the body.

Even if, researchers were to find no support for the claims leveled against HFCS, it is still a heavy sugar, being added in large amounts to virtually every food product on the market. That in itself is alarming.

Type-2 Diabetes

It's essential for people with diabetes to be aware of this sinister ingredient. Diabetics need to monitor their sugar and carbohydrate intake to prevent sugar spikes. HFCS is high on the glycemic index. Most people do not even know what HFCS is; it just blends in with all the other unpronounceable ingredients on the labels of food packages. It's difficult to avoid being hit by a bullet when you can't identify the shooter. It should be noted that HFCS is as sweet as, or sweeter than, sugar. Like sugar, HFCS has no nutritive value. Need I say more?[33]

Fructose is processed by the liver. When an excessive amount of fructose enters the liver, our bodies produce triglycerides, also known as fats. When fats assimilate within cells, this process causes these cells to become insulin-resistant. This is where diabetes comes in.

Some diabetic dangers of HFCS include:

- A higher consumption of calories
- Excessive consumption of processed foods due to a false sense of hunger
- An increase in body mass
- A possible increase in triglycerides
- Liver Damage

A 2010 research study conducted by Duke University Medical Center concluded that people with a high consumption of HFCS-containing products are at high risk for liver damage in the form of fibrosis, or scarring of the liver. The proper term for this fatal condition is non-alcoholic fatty liver disease (NAFLD). NAFLD can turn into cirrhosis if the scarring is extensive. Cirrhosis is a serious medical condition in which blood flow and liver function become disrupted. Serious consequences can result such as portal hypertension, liver failure, and liver cancer.

Mercury Poisoning

A 2009 study carried out by the Minneapolis-based Institute for Agriculture and Trade Policy (IATP) revealed measurable levels of mercury in 17 out of 55 products tested that contained HFCS. What is the source of this mercury contamination? Industry makers of HFCS use a mercury-containing caustic soda to separate corn starch from the corn kernel. Caustic soda is a strong alkali manufactured in (chlor-alkali) industrial chlorine plants where mercury is used; thus, HFCS is susceptible to contamination. The **Food and Drug Administration** may have known about this contamination for years. I can tell you there is no acceptable level of mercury in the food I eat.[34, 35, 36]

Medical studies have attributed mercury poisoning to the following illnesses:

Acrodynia

Fibromyalgia

Alzheimer's

Intestinal Dysfunction

Anterior Lateral Sclerosis (ALS)

Immune System Disorders

Asthma

Kidney Disease

Arthritis	Learning Disorders
Autism	Liver Disorders
Candida	Lupus
Cardiovascular Disease	Metabolic Encephalopathy
Chronic Fatigue Syndrome	Multiple Sclerosis (MS)
Crohn's Disease	Reproductive Disorders
Depression	Parkinson's Disease
Developmental Defects	Senile Dementia
Diabetes	Thyroid Disease
Hormonal Dysfunction	

Aspartame

Aspartame goes under several brand names including NutraSweet, Equal, Equal-Measure, and Spoonful. Chemist James Schlatter of the G.D. Searle Company accidentally discovered aspartame during the testing of an anti-ulcer drug. Aspartame received approval for use in dry goods in 1974; final approval was withheld until 1981, due to an FDA investigation into G.D. Searle's research practices. Aspartame was introduced to the carbonated beverages market in 1983.[37]

Aspartame is the biggest contributor to the FDA's Reportable Food Registry concerning potentially harmful reactions caused by food additives. A number of studies have associated heavy ingestion of aspartame with the following health conditions:

Alzheimer's Disease	Hormonal Problems
Anterior Lateral Sclerosis (ALS)	Hypoglycemia
Brain Lesions	Memory Loss
Dementia	Multiple Sclerosis (MS)
Epilepsy	Neuroendocrine Disorders
Hearing Loss	Parkinson's Disease

Aspartame is a dipeptide made of the amino acids, aspartic acid, and phenylalanine, and is one of a class of compounds referred to as, "excitotoxins", due to the way in which they "excite" the neurons into action. Aspartame and glutamate are neurotransmitters. When the body exceeds its aspartame or glutamate limit, a surplus of calcium builds up in the cells. As a result, the amount of free radicals increases, which ultimately leads to the death of the cells.

The blood-brain barrier, which is the separation between the blood and spinal fluid, is a gatekeeper, allowing necessary substances into the brain, while keeping out harmful ones. Aspartic acid and glutamate do not easily pass through the blood-brain barrier.

However, when there is a surplus of these chemicals, they manage to circumvent the system by diffusing into the brain. In the developing brain of a child, this is a recipe for disaster. This circumstance leads to many of the early childhood diseases with which we are all too familiar. There are mechanisms in place that make this happen. If you took the usual high school classes, you might appreciate the science behind this. All you really need to know, is that aspartame can cause serious problems for your body.

At one time, I was drinking up to six cans of diet soda a day. I was lucky if I drank a single glass of water. I just didn't like water because I felt it had no flavor. My sugar addiction didn't help either. My diet soda habit and lack of hydration left me feeling run down. My quality of life was severely impaired. I was irritable, lethargic, and often experienced an upset stomach. This went on for quite some time, until finally I realized what I was doing. As soon as I gave up the diet soda, I opted to replace it with water. Within a short time, I began to feel revitalized. I had more energy and my thinking became clearer too. There are probably millions of chronically dehydrated people in the world, for reasons other than illness. Just to be clear, overconsumption of aspartame can most certainly be a strong contributing factor to dehydration. I can personally attest to this statement.

Monosodium Glutamate

In 1907, a Japanese scientist named Kikunae Ikeda discovered glutamic acid while researching the flavor-enhancing qualities of seaweed. Ikeda named this distinct quality of MSG "unami." A patent for mass-producing MSG soon followed Kikune's infamous discovery.[38]

MSG is the sodium salt of an amino acid called glutamic acid (glutamate). We know that amino acids link together to form proteins, and, therefore, are the "building blocks of life." The body manufactures some aminos, while others come from the foods we eat. Proteins play a pivotal role in such things as:

- The arrangement or formation of the tissues, organs, and other parts of the body

- Chemical messengers that are produced in the body which have specific regulatory functions in the activity of certain cells and organs

- Enzymes, which are protein molecules that speed up chemical reactions in the body

- Hormones, which are chemicals, typically a peptide or steroid that carries messages from the organs of your body to your cells, and affect such things as growth and metabolism

Amino acids not used up immediately, undergo certain metabolic processes to be converted into fuel, which will be stored for later use. The body converts the amino acid salt aspartate into glutamate. If an excessive amount of aspartate enters the body, illness can result.

Free glutamic acid is processed using hydrolyzing vegetable protein or autolyzed yeast extract. Foods that naturally contain MSG are not a problem. However, MSG added to foods can be harmful. Supporters of MSG claim, it is okay in any form, since it occurs naturally in the body. However, MSG is markedly different from its natural cousin because of the manner in which it is processed. They are not equal.

Some of you might be wondering what purpose MSG serves. MSG is a food additive that enhances flavor. It stimulates the receptors of the taste buds; making our body perceive the food we eat to seem especially savory, and, therefore, more appetizing. Aspartate and glutamate stimulate the same receptor cells (nerve endings that respond to sensory stimuli). Therefore MSG changes the way food tastes and our opinion of it. In a way, it changes your personal reality. At least it changes the reality of what you are eating. Maybe I'm carrying this a little too far, but I believe it's a interesting idea.

The glutamate in MSG stimulates the pancreas to excrete insulin. This should be of concern to us, since a lack of carbohydrates leaves the body with nothing to manage. Of course, when we crash from a drop in blood sugar, we get hungry. What an ideal situation for the manufacturers using MSG in their food products.

There have been numerous reports made to the FDA about the side effects of MSG. Some of common complaints include:

- Headache, sometimes called an MSG headache
- Flushing
- Sweating
- Sense of facial pressure or tightness
- Numbness, tingling, or burning in, or, around the mouth
- Rapid, fluttering heartbeats (heart palpitations)
- Chest pain
- Shortness of breath
- Nausea
- Weakness

Obesity is but one of the dangerous health conditions that can be attributed to MSG. Dr. Russell Blaylock, the neurosurgeon and author who is famous for his denouncement of both aspartame and MSG, states that the following side effects can be experienced through the consumption of MSG:

- Seizures
- Brain cell death
- Brain damage
- Allergies
- Headaches
- Strokes
- Hypoglycemia
- Brain Tumors

You will find MSG in the following ingredients:

Autolyzed yeast	Monosodium glutamate
Calcium caseinate	Monopotassium glutamate
Gelatin	Natrium glutamate
Glutamate	Sodium caseinate
Glutamic acid	Textured protein
Hydrolyzed protein	Yeast extract
Hydrolyzed corn gluten	Yeast food

Yeast nutrient

The following contain or use MSG or MSG in the processing:

Anything fermented	Natural flavor(s)
Anything enzyme modified	Natural pork flavoring
Enzymes anything	Pectin
Anything soy fortified	Protease
Barley malt	Protein enzymes
Bouillon & broth	Seasoning
Carrageenan	Soy protein
Citric acid	Soy protein isolate
Flavor(s) & flavoring(s)	Soy sauce
Malt extract	Soy sauce extract
Malt flavoring	Soy protein concentrate
Maltodextrin	Ultra-pasteurized
Natural chicken flavoring	Whey protein

Natural beef flavoring   Whey protein concentrate

Whey protein isolate

Researchers estimate that up to a quarter of Americans may be allergic, intolerant, or sensitive to MSG. Reactions can lead to rashes, bowel urgencies, headaches, tachycardia, and in some instances depression. I can speak to this issue, on behalf of a friend who once fell unconscious at a Chinese restaurant some years ago. After being closely examined in the emergency room, doctors advised my friend he had experienced an allergic reaction to MSG.[39, 40]

Trans-Fatty Acids

In the late 1800s, Nobel laureate Paul Sabatier developed the process for hydrogenation. While Sabatier was able to perfect hydrogenation of vapors, in 1902, German chemist Wilhelm Normann received a patent for the hydrogenation of oils. Normann's process used hydrogen to convert double bonds in the molecules of vegetable oil into single bonds. This chemical conversion results in the formation of trans-fats, which are, in fact, very similar to saturated fats. For example, unsaturated cottonseed oil when hydrogenated forms solid fats.

Proctor and Gamble saw the profitability in this new technique and purchased the patent from Normann in 1911. Shortly thereafter, Crisco was conceived and unleashed on uninformed consumers. Crisco comes in part from hydrogenated cottonseed oil.

After an outcry in the mid-1980s by public interest groups, the fast food industry switched to using trans-fats rather than saturated fats. This trend changed in 2006, when the American Heart

Association specified that daily consumption of trans-fats, should account for less than one percent of total calories consumed. It was also in that year that New York passed a law limiting trans-fats in restaurants; followed in 2008 by a unanimous vote of the Boston Public Health Commission to ban trans-fats in Boston city restaurants. The controversy continues as the momentum against trans-fat builds.

Food manufacturers are fond of trans-fats because of the long shelf life they can achieve by adding it to their food products, and we're paying for it, in more ways than one. Simply stated, it's healthy for their profit margin and unhealthy for our bodies.[41]

Besides shortening and margarine, trans-fats are contained in these foods:

Biscuits	French fries
Cake	Fried Chicken
Cake icing	Fried fish
Candy	Microwave popcorn
Cereals	Muffins
Cookies	Pie
Crackers	Salad Dressings
Donuts	Waffles

Trans-fatty acids increase the blood levels of bad low-density lipoprotein (LDL) cholesterol, while at the same time lowering good, high-density lipoprotein (HDL) cholesterol. This makes trans-fats much more harmful to our bodies than saturated fat, which has largely replaced trans-fats in processed products such as baked goods. This situation increases your risk of heart disease. The Center for Disease Control and Prevention (CDC) currently maintains this alarming statement on their website (www.cdc.gov/features/heartmonth) regarding heart disease,

"Heart disease is the leading cause of death in the United States and is a leading cause of disability. The most common heart disease in the United States is coronary heart disease, which often appears as a heart attack. In 2009, an estimated 785,000 Americans had a new coronary attack, and about 470,000 will have a recurrent attack. About every 25 seconds, an American will have a coronary event, and about one every minute will die from one."[42]

Some studies have linked trans-fatty acids to Alzheimer's disease and cancer:

Alzheimer's Disease

In February of 2003, *The Archives of Neurology* included an article entitled "Dietary Fats and the Risk of Incident Alzheimer's disease." The article summarizes the findings of a study, which followed the eating habits of 815 mentally healthy senior citizens. The study concluded that there is a correlation between both saturated fats and trans-fats, and the elevated risk of developing Alzheimer's disease. The study revealed that the participants who were in the highest 80% trans-fat consumption level were four times as likely to develop Alzheimer's as the lowest 20%, who consumed

188

approximately 1.8 grams of trans fat on average. The study also showed that a diet high in trans-fat, and low in polyunsaturated fat make a person nine times more at risk of developing Alzheimer's, than a person maintaining a diet low in trans-fat and high in polyunsaturated fat.

Alzheimer's disease is the most common form of dementia. Alzheimer's destroys neurons responsible for memory and thinking. This affects quality of life. Since it is a progressive brain disease, the symptoms of this illness only go in one direction; bad to worse. A person with Alzheimer's is almost certain to die sooner rather than later. In fact, Alzheimer's is the seventh leading cause of death in the US. The National Institute on Aging estimates there are between 2.4 million and 4.5 million Americans with Alzheimer's. There is no known medical cure for this devastating illness.[43, 44]

Cancer

A recently published study by Harvard establishes a link between trans-fatty acids and prostate cancer. The study followed 15,000 men over thirteen years. Researchers observed an increased risk of non-aggressive prostate tumors by monitoring the intake of trans-isomers of oleic, and linoleic acids.[45]

About the Author

David Almeida is a Certified Hypnotist. He was a successful Licensed Private Investigator for over 20 years. His areas of practice included criminal defense, domestic investigations, missing persons, background checks, and fraud. David received the admiration of his corporate and notable clients for his behind the scenes work on their sensitive cases. He completed hundreds of diverse cases during his distinguished career. David considers himself an "intuitive investigator." He used his uncanny intuitive sense to solve his most difficult cases. While David values his professional experience, he seeks to contribute to the betterment of society by helping others awaken to their true spiritual potential. His curiosity compels him to peer into the unknown searching for lost metaphysical knowledge. David maintains a fulfilling and meaningful life with his wife of 18 years and spunky Jack Russell Terrier.

Inquiries: davidalmeida@usa.com

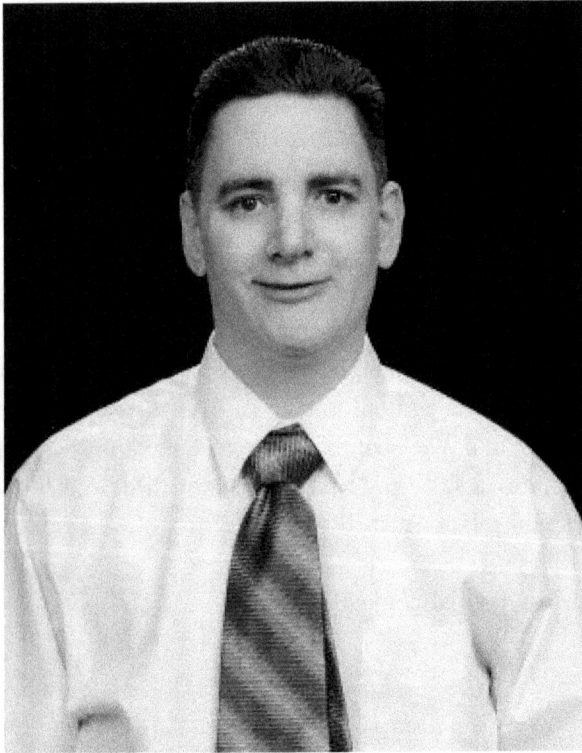

David Almeida

Index

End Notes

[1] Peter Tomkins and Christopher Bird, *The Secret Life of Plants*. (New York, NY: Harper and Row, 1973, 344-56.

[2] Wikipedia, *George De La Warr*, http://en.wikipedia.org/wiki/George_de_la_Warr, February 16, 2011.

[3] World Research Foundation, *The Electrical Patterns of Life; The Work of Dr. Harold S. Burr*, http://www.wrf.org/men-women-medicine/dr-harold-s-burr.php, August 1, 2010.

[4] Ronald E. Matthews, *Harold Burr's Biofields - Measuring the Electromagnetics of Life*, The Energy Medicine Institute, http://www.energymed.org/hbank/handouts/harold_burr_biofields.htm, August 1, 2010.

[5] Tomkins and Bird, 82-103.

[6] India Guide, *Jagadish Chandra Bose Biography*, http://www.iloveindia.com/indian-heroes/jagadish-chandra-bose.html, August 25, 2010.

[7] Incredible People, Biography of Jagadish Chandra Bose, profiles.incredible-people.com/jagadish-chandra-bose, August 10, 2010.

[8] Tomkins and Bird, *ibid.*

[9] Answers.com, *Cleve Backster*, http://www.answers.com/topic/cleve-backster, September 5, 2010.

[10] Cleve Backster, "Evidence of a Primary Perception in Plant Life," *International Journal of Parapsychology* 10 (4), 1968: 329-348.

[11] Cherry Kendra, *The Science of Love: Harry Harlow and the Nature of Affection*, http://psychology.about.com/od/historyofpsychology/p/harlow_love.htm, September 18, 2010.

[12] Lothar Wolff, "Rock a Bye Baby," (1970), http://www.violence.de/tv/rockabye.html, September 18, 2010.

[13] University of Wisconsin, *The Science of Mother's Day*, http://whyfiles.org/087mother/4.html, September 22, 2010.

[14] Peter Groen, David Levine, and Douglas Goldstein, *Complementary and Alternative Medicine (CAM) and Electronic Health Record (EHR) Systems*, http://www.hoise.com/vmw/06/articles/vmw/LV-VM-03-06-11.html, October 1, 2010.

[15] Dr. Ken Duckworth, *Transcranial Magnetic Stimulation (TMS Or rTMS*, http://www.nami.org/Content/ContentGroups/Helpline1/Transcranial_Magnetic_Stimulation_(rTMS).htm, *October 14, 2010.*

[16] Sarah H. Lisanby, Bruce Luber, Tarique Perera, and Harold A. Sackiem, *Trancranial magnetic Stimulation: Applications in Basic Neuroscience and Neuropsychopharmcology*, http://www.contemporarycare.net/uploads/documents/TMSReviewPerera.pdf, 2000.

[17] Medical university of South Carolina, *Brain-Stimulation Method Appears to Help Induce Remission in Some Patients with Depression*, http://www.musc.edu/pr/brain_stimulation.htm, *May 3, 2010.*

[18] The School for New Learning, DePaul University, *Transcendentalism*, http://condor.depaul.edu/dsimpson/awtech/amertran.html, November 29, 2010.

[19] Donna M. Campbell, *American Transcendentalism* - adapted from *Resisting Regionalism: Gender and Naturalism in American Fiction, 1885-1915* (Athens: Ohio University Press, 1997), http://public.wsu.edu/~campbelld/amlit/amtrans.htm, March 21, 2010.

[20] Robert D. Richardson, Jr. from *Emerson: The Mind on Fire, The Transcendental Club,* http://www.vcu.edu/engweb/ transcendentalism/ideas/club.html, November 29, 2010.

[21] http://www.tm.org/

[22] AllExperts Questions and Answers, *Anorexia/Eating Disorders,* http://en.allexperts.com/q/Anorexia-Eating-Disorders-1604/anorexia, December 2, 2010.

[23] Mental Health Information and Resource Directory, *Anorexia and Bulimia,* http://www.outreach-online.org/leaflets/anorexiaBulimia/ anorexiaBulimia.htm, December 2, 2010.

[24] Melinda Smith, Sarah Kovatch, and Jeanne Segal, *Anorexia Nervosa: Signs, Symptoms, Causes, and Treatment,* http://www.helpguide.org/mental/anorexia_signs_symptoms_causes_ treatment.htm, December 3, 2010.

[25] The Cleveland Clinic Foundation, Munchausen Syndrome, http://my.clevelandclinic.org/disorders/factitious_disorders/hic_munc hausen_syndrome.aspx, December 10, 2010.

[26] Chris, Simpson, *Self-Mutilation,* http://www.athealth.com/ Consumer/disorders/selfmutilation.html, December 18, 2010.

[27] SixWise.com, *The Dangers of Nitrites: The Foods They Are Found in and Why You Want to Avoid Them,* http://www.sixwise.com/newsletters/ 07/08/22/the-dangers-of- nitrites-the-foods-they-are-found-in-and-why-you-want-to-avoid- them.htm, December 27, 2010.

[28] Jane Ann Boles and Ronald Pegg, *Meat Color,* http://animalrange.montana.edu/courses/meat/meatcol.pdf, December 27, 2010.

[29] Science of Cooking, *What is the Difference between Nitrites and Nitrates,* http://www.scienceofcooking.com/nitrites_and_nitrates.htm, December 27, 2010.

[30] Miranda Hitti, *Study: Cured Meats, COPD May Be Linked*, http://www.webmd.com/news/20070417/study-copd-cured-meats-may-be-linked, December 28, 2010.

[31] Global Healing Center, *5 Health Dangers of High Fructose Corn Syrup,* http://www.globalhealingcenter.com/natural-health/high-fructose-corn-syrup-dangers, December 30, 2010.

[32] Living a Healthy Lifestyle, *Dangerous Food Ingredients Are Contributing to Obesity and Cancer*, http://www.living-a-healthy-lifestyle.com/dangerous-food-ingredients.html, January 1, 2011.

[33] Christopher R. Mohr, *The Dangers of High Fructose Corn Syrup*, http://www.diabeteshealth.com/read/2008/08/20/4274/the-dangers-of-high-fructose-corn-syrup, January 1, 2011.

[34] Miranda Hitti, *Researchers Say 17 Products Tested Had Some Mercury; Industry Group Says Syrup Is Safe*, http://www.webmd.com/food-recipes/news/20090127/mercury-in-high-fructose-corn-syrup, January 3, 2011.

[35] Leslie Hatfield, *Our Melamine: There's Mercury in High Fructose Corn Syrup, and the FDA Has Known for Years*, http://www.huffingtonpost.com/leslie-hatfield/our-melamine-theres-mercu_b_161334.html, January 3, 2011.

[36] Christian Goodman, *High Fructose Corn Syrup Causes High blood Pressure*, http://ezinearticles.com/?High-Fructose-Corn-Syrup-Causes-High-Blood-Pressure&id=3445941, January 4, 2011.

[37] Dr. Joseph Mercola, *Aspartame: What You Don't Know Can Hurt You,* http://aspartame.mercola.com, January 5, 2011.

[38] Will Levine and edited by Heather Kelley, *MSG: Its history, effects and what you can do to avoid it*, http://www.foodconsumer.org/newsite/Safety/chemical/22042009044

8_msg_its_history_effects_and_what_you_can_do_to_avoi.html, January 8, 2011.

[39] Gregory Paul Johnson, *Monosodium Glutamate MSG Health Dangers and Side Effects of Toxic Additives*, http://www.resourcesforlife.com/docs/item1225, January 9, 2011.

[40] Living-A-Healthy-Lifesyle.com, *Dangerous Food Ingredients Are Contributing to Obesity and Cancer*, http://www.living-a-healthy-lifestyle.com/dangerous-food-ingredients.html, January 9, 2011.

[41] Dangerous Food Ingredients Are Contributing to Obesity and Cancer, ibid.

[42] Centers for Disease Control and Prevention, *February Is American Heart Month*, http://www.cdc.gov/features/heartmonth, *January 13, 2011.*

[43] TFX, *The Campaign against Trans-Fats in Foods, Trans fats, Alzheimer Disease and Cognitive Decline: The "Dietary Fats and the Risk of Incident Alzheimer Disease" Study*, http://www.tfx.org.uk/page131.html, January 9, 2010.

[44] Alzheimer's Association, *What is Alzheimer's*, http://www.alz.org/alzheimers_disease_what_is_alzheimers.asp, *January 15, 2011.*

[45] Stephen Daniells, *Trans-Fats Harm May Extend to Prostate: Study*, http://www.foodnavigator.com/Science-Nutrition/Trans-fats-harm-may-extend-to-prostate-study, January 15, 2011.

www.ingramcontent.com/pod-product-compliance
Lightning Source LLC
LaVergne TN
LVHW051512080426
835509LV00017B/2043